Evidence-Based Medicine
Best Practice or Restrictive Dogma

Evidence-Based Medicine
Best Practice or Restrictive Dogma

Desmond J Sheridan

Imperial College London, UK

Imperial College Press

ICP

Published by

Imperial College Press
57 Shelton Street
Covent Garden
London WC2H 9HE

Distributed by

World Scientific Publishing Co. Pte. Ltd.

5 Toh Tuck Link, Singapore 596224

USA office: 27 Warren Street, Suite 401-402, Hackensack, NJ 07601

UK office: 57 Shelton Street, Covent Garden, London WC2H 9HE

Library of Congress Cataloging-in-Publication Data
Names: Sheridan, Desmond J. (Desmond John), author.
Title: Evidence-based medicine : best practice or restrictive dogma / Desmond J Sheridan.
Description: [London] ; New Jersey : Imperial College Press, [2016]
Identifiers: LCCN 2015048799 | ISBN 9781783267620 (hc : alk. paper)
Subjects: | MESH: Evidence-Based Medicine
Classification: LCC R723.7 | NLM WB 102.5 | DDC 610--dc23
LC record available at http://lccn.loc.gov/2015048799

British Library Cataloguing-in-Publication Data
A catalogue record for this book is available from the British Library.

Desk Editors: Harini/Mary Simpson

Typeset by Stallion Press
Email: enquiries@stallionpress.com

Printed in Singapore

Lobbying!
Selected truths advance causes,
over-simplifications beguile us,
rhetoric diverts and distracts us.
The Pied Piper of our age!

Preface

In 1991 a group of epidemiologists based at McMaster University launched the concept of Evidence-Based Medicine (EBM), as a new paradigm for medical practice. It rapidly captured the attention of medics, health service managers and the general media. Voted idea of the year by the New York Times in 2001 and short-listed among "medical milestone" by the BMJ in 2007, EBM proved to be one of the most successful medical campaigns in recent history. In this book I have explored the origins and reasons for its remarkable rise and its far reaching impact on clinical medicine and medical science, both positive and adverse; and why its timing was perfectly aligned with events taking place in health service delivery as well as in the funding of medical research.

The book also discusses criticisms of some concepts advocated by the EBM movement; why clinicians and philosophers objected to its notion of a hierarchy of evidence and to its over simplification of the nature of evidence. I argue that some of its tenets are contrary to values doctors must uphold in caring for individual patients and have contributed to problems in healthcare management. The book also examines why the rise of EBM coincided with a decline in clinical science in the UK and how the comparative research on which EBM is based came to replace clinical science with lasting harmful consequences.

Medical practice based on reliable evidence is now a recognised value of medical professionalism, which doctors must uphold in caring for patients.

As such, I argue that EBM is one of several values in medicine and cannot be overriding, for example above the wishes and feelings of patients. In looking to the future, I argue that EBM must be a set of principles which guide medicine widely. It cannot be a movement with a restricted mission or agenda, which ignores important areas that impact on care of patients. The EBM movement has presented itself as fiercely independent of commercial interests in healthcare; however I argue that it has been too closely aligned with political power and the main drivers of the healthcare reforms. Indeed the volume of EBM advocacy has often distracted attention from these areas in even greater need of scrutiny.

In writing this book I am aware that some of my views may meet with disagreement. However if they help to initiate discussions which must take place if EBM is to become a set of principles that guide medicine and healthcare in a meaningful way it will have served a useful purpose.

Contents

Preface   vii

Chapter 1   The Origins of Evidence-Based Medicine   1

Chapter 2   Evidence-Based Medicine in the UK   19

Chapter 3   The Cochrane Collaboration   37

Chapter 4   Evidence-Based Medicine and the Evolution of Health
            Related Research   59

Chapter 5   Hypothesis, Evidence, Knowledge and Reasoning
            in Medicine: Certainty and Uncertainty   95

Chapter 6   Evidenced-Based Medicine and Medical Science   125

Chapter 7   Impact of Evidence-Based Medicine on Clinical
            Practice: Achievements and Limitations   151

Chapter 8   Evidence-Based Medicine and Medical Professionalism   173

Chapter 9   The Future of Evidence-Based Medicine   197

Index   215

Chapter 1

The Origins of Evidence-Based Medicine

The rise of Evidence-Based Medicine, often referred to as EBM, during the last years of the 20th century and early in the 21st has been both rapid and dramatic. Apart from a small number of committed advocates it was unheard of prior to the 1990s but since then it has come to occupy a powerful role in medicine with official backing and sponsorship from governments and strong support within the medical profession itself, as well as many allied professions and lay groups. Along the way EBM has also attracted significant dissent, mainly among philosophers concerned with the concepts and principles behind it, but it has not been short of vociferous defenders and this has led to a lively exchange between detractors and advocates. This discussion has largely been confined to academia, apart from the occasional spill over into the general media. It is without doubt one of the most important developments in medicine during the past half century. What is it and from where did it come?

EBM: Brand New or New Branding?

The term Evidence-Based Medicine was first used in 1991[1] and more formally in 1992.[2] At first reading it appears a fairly innocuous phrase, even a statement of the obvious. What could be controversial about medicine based on evidence? What kind of medicine would be evidence-based? The apparent simplicity of the phrase belied hidden complexities and the far reaching ambitions which its proponents had in mind, which were nothing short of a new approach to the teaching and practicing of medicine. What did it mean? A definition offered in a defence of EBM[3] was as follows, "Evidence-based medicine is the conscientious, explicit, and judicious use of current best evidence in making decisions about the care of individual patients." Again, on first reading there appears to be nothing contentious in this, but then there are the thorny questions of what constitutes evidence, what does it include or exclude and what does it prioritise and relegate. Neither does this definition specify what is meant by "best evidence" nor how and by what means it would be identified. These questions have been at the root of much of the dissent surrounding EBM in the years that followed. But first I will consider EBM in the context of developments in medicine over time. Is EBM new or a rebranding of something which had existed previously?

The title EBM was new in that it had not been in use previously and it gave a new name to the field it represented. It also gave a new impetus for a modernisation that was needed to facilitate and manage the explosion of medical information that had begun in the 1970s. By the late 1970s, it was already becoming clear that new methods were needed to manage the increased volume of scientific information being produced. To illustrate this, Durrack[4] weighed volumes of the Index Medicus, an annual comprehensive list of articles published in medical science journals since 1874. These had been stable for many decades, but doubled in weight between 1946 and 1955 and then increased over seven fold between 1955 and 1977. EBM advocated new ways to teach and practice medicine in a manner that would incorporate this new knowledge. The methods of EBM have been widely published and adopted, although not without controversy. Supporters of EBM have reminded us that it was voted "idea of the year" by the *New York Times* in 2001[5] and considered among a list of medical milestones in a survey carried out by the *British Medical Journal.*[6] The EBM movement, as it came to be known, can therefore reasonably claim to have articulated the need for a new development in medical teaching and practice to reflect the rapid expansion of clinical research and the need to manage and interpret the increased amount of scientific information being published.

However, the idea that the EBM movement had invented a new method of practicing medicine seems less credible when one looks at its development in the context of what preceded it. The need for more efficient management of scientific medical information had already been identified and would become inevitable, given the extraordinary advances which were taking place in computing and communication technology. Credit is due to the EBM movement for its skilled use of rhetoric to capture the agenda and to galvanise the medical community into action sooner than might otherwise have occurred. However, in doing so, there are aspects of the case it made, particularly in relation to its novelty and the methods used which I will argue, were not always justified. Advocates of EBM, in response to critics, have acknowledged that "depending on one's perspective" the origins of EBM extend back centuries.[7] What then is the history of collecting evidence for the purpose of improving medical practice? It is worth looking at this in some detail because some of the adverse reactions to EBM have in my view had as much to do with the manner in which it was presented as the content of the message it embodies. This matters if we are to identify what is valuable in the concept and avoid throwing the baby out with the bathwater.

EBM: The McMaster Model

The story of EBM in our own time took off in 1991 with a paper published from McMaster University,[1] which has often been referred to by subsequent writers as having coined the phrase EBM. This and a subsequent paper,[2] published the following year by authors calling themselves The EBM Group, again mainly based at McMaster, has been highly influential in advocating EBM and I will discuss these two papers in some detail. The 1991 article consisted of a one page editorial which described a case history of possible iron deficiency anaemia investigated by a young internist. The writer invites readers to envisage two scenarios labelled "The way of the past" and "The way of the future". In the former, the internist relies on what she was told by senior colleagues during earlier training and proceeds accordingly. In the latter, she refers immediately to the literature to obtain information about relevant tests in making the diagnosis. In the process she discovers that what she was told during training conflicts with the literature and that her laboratory's normal range for the test is misleading. She estimates a pre-test probability of iron deficiency anaemia (based on published information about the prevalence of the illness in a group of patients with similar clinical features) and orders the test. She then calculates the post-test probability of iron deficiency anaemia based on published information about the sensitivity (how good it is in identifying cases) and specificity (how good it is at identifying only real cases and avoiding misdiagnosing people with or without the illness) of the test, and manages the case accordingly.

The article then used the scenarios to describe "the way of the past" as one in which clinicians looked solely to what it referred to as "authority" for information and guidance regarding patient management. In contrast "the way of the future", called EBM, would involve clinicians quickly searching the literature to obtain relevant information to guide clinical management. In order to practice EBM, clinicians would need to learn skills in literature retrieval and evaluation as well as the applicability of information obtained to their patients. The page on which the article appeared even included an advert for the journal as being primarily intended to further EBM.

The essence of the case therefore was that evidence based on the experience and the opinion of colleagues including those in senior positions may be unreliable. Information derived directly from the literature is superior for patient management and clinicians need to learn the skills to do so. This seems fairly obvious today, but given the rapid expansion of clinical research during the preceding decades it was undoubtedly worth emphasising at the time. It is not difficult to see where the seeds of dissent would come from when one looks at the way the article relied so heavily on rhetorical methods to sell what is in effect an important and valuable message. The author's choice of rhetoric, skilfully constructed but rather crudely directed in order to make the case for EBM was bound to attract dissent.

A more formal announcement of EBM was made in a follow-up article in 1992[2] written by what had then become The EBM Working Group. This consisted of 32 members, of whom 24 were affiliated to McMaster University including the author of the 1991 editorial who was its chairman. The predominant specialism among the group was clinical epidemiology. The paper began by announcing that a new paradigm for medical practice was emerging which de-emphasised what it described as intuition, unsystematic clinical experience and pathophysiology as sufficient rationale for clinical decision making, stressing instead the examination of evidence from clinical research.

It then repeated the fictional clinical scenarios used in the 1991 paper to illustrate "the way of the past" and "the way of the future" and invited readers to compare seeking advice from a senior colleague with the use of the literature to make an informed decision. Once again, the unfortunate senior colleagues consulted, were in conflict with the evidence obtained from the literature and the young internist was able avoid being misled by going independently to primary sources of information in the literature.

It is not difficult to envisage why this rhetorical approach might have irritated some clinicians who would fall into the "senior colleague" category. Some might not unreasonably have felt that they were being consigned to the dustbin of history. Later in the paper the EBM group did acknowledge a role for clinical skills, an understanding of pathophysiology, compassion and sensitivity to the emotional needs of patients. However, the fundamental concept advocated by the group was the idea of a hierarchy of evidence in medicine, with randomised controlled trials at the top and all other forms of evidence being of lesser quality and reliability. The teaching of traditional clinical skills was to be provided by clinicians, but under the guidance of experts trained in EBM as minders to ensure the "way of the future" was correctly taught. In this way students would learn how to "precisely define a patient problem" and "what information is required to resolve it". This was to be called "critical appraisal" and was something the group considered had not been part of traditional teaching methods.

The paper then described the medical curriculum at McMaster University Department of Medicine which the authors judged to be the strongest in teaching EBM although no evidence or other information was presented as to how this was arrived at. The main features of this program are outlined in Box 1.1. The inclusion of specific time to teach students how to access and evaluate published literature may not have been widely included in curricula at the time and its emphasis would have been helpful. Stressing the need for communication technology to provide access to the literature once again was helpful. However, the notion that an intransigent medical establishment was resisting this is hardly justified when one looks at the speed with which communication technology has been widely adopted in medicine, which seems hardly less swift than in other areas of education. In practice, this was evolving widely at the time, but not in the way advocated. To be effective, these systems needed to be available to groups of students and

---

Box 1.1   The EBM Program at McMaster.[2]

1. A weekly afternoon devoted to teaching reliable methods for interpreting published articles related to diagnosis and treatment and discussion of clinical cases and relevant literature.
2. Facilities for literature searching made available on teaching wards to access relevant information immediately.
3. Candidates who had received training in clinical epidemiology were appointed to the Dept. of Medicine, because it was argued, such individuals "have the skills and commitment to practice EBM". The residency program also worked to ensure that teaching roles were made available to them.
4. Rigorous evaluation of attending physicians' effectiveness in teaching EBM was instituted.
5. Attending physicians were encouraged to form partnerships to attend each other's rounds and provide observations and feedback.
6. Attending physicians were required to be "enthusiastic and effective" role models for the practice of EBM.
7. Training in clinical skills provided by clinicians with guidance from experts in EBM.

---

in practice they were implemented most widely in hospital library facilities. I suspect that for most practicing clinicians the idea of interrupting, for example, the clinical assessment of a patient while teaching or during rounds in order to undertake immediate literature searches would not be considered helpful. Furthermore, while some patients might understand its purpose, others might feel it diminished their experience of the consultation and their emotional needs. It also underestimates the ability of students to capture the questions and uncertainties that arise on the ward and to investigate them later. In any event, technology has moved on and most students these days have personal portable devices which can provide all of this technology.

Clinical epidemiology is undoubtedly an essential specialism in medicine, however, the EBM group did not set out any evidence to support its belief that this expertise uniquely provides the "skills and commitment" to practice EBM as distinct from any other. The group itself was composed mostly of epidemiologists, which poses a risk of bias in favour of an exclusive and self-promoting logic. If I am a clinical epidemiologist, and I believe that EBM is the future of medicine, and that only clinical epidemiologists holding similar beliefs to mine can teach EBM, then only my views can succeed and all other avenues are excluded. This would seem contrary to a meaningful and one might add evidence based debate within the faculty and to restrict avenues for development.

Evaluation and appraisal of physicians have developed markedly during the past two decades. This applies to teaching as well as practice and is broadly welcomed as a good thing. However, the focus on rigorous assessment of physicians' effectiveness in teaching EBM seems premature when the group's vision of EBM itself had not been evaluated. There is the question of who would do the evaluation and on what grounds would physicians be assessed? Would for example a commitment to the beliefs espoused by the EBM group be important? And would this include the group's vision of how the curriculum should be managed, staffed and organised?

Attending physicians were encouraged to form partnerships to attend each other's rounds and provide observations and feedback. This is in fact a long standing and well established practice in most clinical settings, but perhaps not with the frequency and intensity implied by the EBM group.

The requirement that attending physicians should be "enthusiastic and effective" role models for the practice of EBM raises questions as to how this would be assessed and what the assessment would entail. While the fundamental idea of teaching students on how to evaluate the biomedical literature is undeniable, the EBM group went far beyond this in advocating a vision of how medical practice and teaching should be organised and managed based on an exclusive and untested model.

Emphasising to students the importance and value of searching the literature to improve clinical decision making, which the authors call "critical appraisal" is helpful. But again the principal here is in fact widely accepted and practiced.

In advocating their vision, the EBM, group argued that EBM represented a new paradigm in medical teaching and practice,[2] based on its idea of a hierarchy of evidence for guiding medical practice with published randomised controlled trials at the top. This it was argued was so new and profound that it made the existing model untenable. While it would be true to say that a model of clinical practice which ignored the literature would indeed be untenable, this was hardly a reasonable judgement of the existing model of practice. After all it was the existing model which produced the rapid expansion of the biomedical literature during the preceding decades and created the material on which EBM was to be built. Furthermore, it seems inconceivable that this extraordinary expansion of knowledge could have occurred in a model of clinical medicine which was as divorced from the literature as implied by the EBM group. In reality, the claim that EBM represented a paradigm shift could only stand if past efforts to base medicine on evidence were discounted and this appears to be implicit in the rhetoric used by the group. No evidence was provided to support such a claim other than the fictional clinical scenarios to discount the "way of the past". This was coupled with what looks like a systematic avoidance of acknowledging any previous efforts to establish medicine on a rational and evidence base.

The EBM group did acknowledge that objections to its vision, which it attributed to misapprehensions about EBM, had arisen and sought to correct these.[2] This took the form of "correcting" three misinterpretations, namely that (a) EBM ignores clinical expertise and intuition, (b) that understanding basic investigation and pathophysiology plays no part in EBM and (c) that EBM ignores standard aspects of clinical training such as clinical examination. In response to these allegations, the group clarified that all of these would in fact remain essential elements of clinical training and practice. This of course did not address the most important objection to the views put forward by the EBM group; namely, whether a real hierarchy of evidence based on its quality and reliability is justified and appropriate for managing clinical encounters.

Thus, the essence of EBM as envisioned by McMaster group was a hierarchy of evidence with literature retrieval to identify objective reliable information at the top; evidence-based on opinion, experience and authority being of lesser quality and possibly unreliable and possibly misleading. The value of randomised controlled trials and methods of literature retrieval had already been recognised and were advancing rapidly. What proved more contentious were the tactics and rhetoric used by the group to advocate and spread their views. The claim to have discovered and implemented a new paradigm of clinical teaching and practice was to say the least extravagant. The use of over, simplified fictional clinical scenarios to promote the desired vision of the future by casting the past in a poor light might have seemed justified to a group with strongly held views. It was certainly provocative and succeeded in capturing attention. But it also tended to undermine the vision being advocated in that it exemplified the very thing it sought to change, namely action on the basis of rhetoric rather than evidence.

The manner in which EBM was delivered at McMaster was unusual in the extent to which the role played by staff trained in clinical epidemiology was emphasised. Clinical epidemiologists undoubtedly play an essential role in medicine and public health. However, as discussed above their central role in the EBM group, in advocating its vision and in the organisation and delivery of EBM appears exclusive and self-promoting, more in keeping with a committed activist approach than seeking change though rational discourse. A striking feature of the EBM group was its failure to acknowledge earlier workers in promoting the use of objective evidence in clinical practice. This may have reflected an attempt to focus on improving the future rather than rehearsing the past. However, it has the appearance of an attempt to claim an exclusive mandate for promoting the field, which is unfortunate in that it distracts from its central message they sought to advocate. In reality, there has been a long standing interest in this area.

Efforts to Build Medicine Based on Evidence from the 18th Century

Interest in objective observation and numerical data collection in medicine was evident early in the 18th century. In order to illustrate this, I will use some examples. For a more detailed account of the history of efforts to improve evidence in medicine, see Trohler.[8] Francis Clifton, a successful London based Physician who trained in Leyden, was concerned that medical practice in his time was based too much on theory, fashion and authority and that his contemporaries were over-prescribing remedies. He wrote two books, "Tabular observations recommended as the plainest and surest way of practising and improving physic",[9] published in 1731 and "The state of physick, ancient and modern, briefly considered: with a plan for the improvement of it"[10] in 1732, which set out his vision of how to improve clinical practice by basing it on sound evidence. In these, Clifton recommended the collection of regular recordings of clinical observations in table form and he proposed a scheme for standardising such tables and the use of short-hand to simplify data entry. He was also aware of the need to control for the subjective assessments of clinicians, and recommended the employment of a person not involved in the clinical management of the patients concerned. His aim was to put clinical decision making on a more objective basis, rather than on modern fashions. Clifton died relatively young in Jamaica in 1736 where he was preparing an account of the diseases on the island. It is remarkable how closely Clifton's concerns about the practice of medicine and the principals he advocated for improving it mirror those promoted in our own times. However, unlike some of his modern successors he believed that answers to the challenges he identified were to be found in classical learning.

John Clark (1744–1805), while a surgeon on a sailing ship of the East India Company from 1768 to 1772, kept a register of the cases he treated. On the basis of his systematic observations he became aware of the adverse effects of "copious bleeding" which was recommended for treating fevers at the time. As a result, he decided to use instead Peruvian cinchona bark and published his results in 1773.[11] He was careful to present a detailed account of his cases including deaths and unsuccessful treatments in order to provide a reliable evaluation of his method. He later compared mortality on seven ships in which no bark was given with his own results. On returning to England he set up a dispensary in Newcastle upon Tyne where he continued his practice of carefully recording details of his cases. In 1780, he published records for all cases seen between October 1st 1777 and October 1st 1779.[12] During the two years concerned he treated 743 patients of whom 48 died. These included 6 deaths among 203 cases of "continued fevers", 6 deaths in 30 cases of small pox and 13 in 95 cases of scarlet fever. He also included a detailed account of all who died. Clark was aware of the value of systematic recording of all cases in order to accurately assess the value of treatments and he was critical of the haphazard accounts which had been common at the time. In a later book published in 1792,[13] he brought together cases he had seen in Newcastle upon Tyne and those he had cared for earlier at sea. He also arranged to collect all of the cases recorded on ships of the East India Company from 1770 to 1785. He could see that such careful recording of cases, their treatment and outcomes would serve to identify optimal therapy and save lives.

The importance of systematic comparison of treatments was also advocated by Edward Alanson (1747–1823) who studied under John Hunter in

London. Alanson was appointed to the Liverpool Infirmary in 1770 and was a meticulous record keeper throughout his career. He was one of the earliest surgeons to introduce immediate closure of amputation wounds rather than relying on healing by secondary intention. He was concerned that changing the practice of such a serious operation, which he described in the preface to his 1782 book[14] as "terrible to bear, horrid to see, and must leave the person on whom it has been performed, in a mutilated imperfect state", should be soundly based. To provide evidence of the superiority of the new method he published a comparison of his results with previous outcomes in 1782.[14] His results clearly showed that leaving an adequate skin flap to allow immediate closure was superior; none of the 35 patients treated by primary closure died compared with 10 of 46 treated by the traditional method. However, he was aware of the limitations of the historical comparison he undertook, regretting that he omitted to take "an accurate history of every amputation, at which I have been present". He was also aware of the potential impact of case selection on outcomes and insisted that all of the 35 cases treated by the new method had been unselected referrals to his hospital practice.

The importance of case selection was also recognised by William Cheselden (1688–1752) who was a noted lithotomy surgeon. He was a skilled anatomist and teacher having trained under William Couper and was appointed surgeon at St Thomas' hospital in 1719. It was there that he became increasingly interested in surgery for bladder stones. He describes his experience of this in Chapter 6 of his 1740 book on human anatomy.[15] The traditional approach for this operation had been *via* a supra pubic route, but after some initial successes Cheselden became disillusioned with it after a number of his patients died. He subsequently tried a perineal approach, which proved more reliable. In recording his results he was aware that patients' characteristics could have an impact on outcomes. He noted that of the 213 operations carried out and witnessed at St Thomas Hospital, of the first 50, 3 died, of the second 50, 3 also died. Eight of the third 50 died and 6 of the last 63 (p. 332). He attributed this to the increasing popularity of the operation and the resulting increasing severity of the cases that were referred to him. He drew particular attention to the important impact which age had on outcomes and he presented his cases in 10-year age groups to demonstrate this. At that time the usual practice was to present crude mortality data. Cheselden's more detailed method changed this as surgeons understood that it provided not only a more reliable analysis of results, but could also be useful in protecting reputations of surgeons following well-publicised case fatalities.

James Lind (1716–1794) trained at the Edinburgh College of Surgeons before working as a ship's doctor from 1739 to 1747. While working on HMS Salisbury he conducted a trial of 6 treatments for scurvy. He was careful to ensure that all of his subjects were at a similar stage of the disease and that they were accommodated in similar conditions.[16] By comparing contemporaneous treatments he demonstrated how the limitations of historical comparisons, which Cheselden had recognised, could be overcome. This was an important step in avoiding selection bias in comparing treatments.

William Withering (1741–1799) trained at Edinburgh and practiced initially at Stafford. In 1775, he was appointed to the Birmingham General Hospital and joined the Lunar Society, both at the behest of Erasmus Darwin. Withering became familiar with the use of foxglove to treat heart failure and over a period of several years developed a reliable dosing scheme. In 1885, he wrote his classic book "Account of the Foxglove and some of its Medical Uses with Practical Remarks on Dropsy and other Diseases".[17] In doing so he identified a number of additional factors which can confound accurate evaluation of medicines. He was concerned that the use of foxglove was becoming popular and he decided to publish his experience of it to avoid its inappropriate use. Withering described 186 cases he treated between 1775 and 1785 and in the preface he noted the necessity to report all his cases rather than a selection of successful ones in order to give a fair and balanced account of the drugs' efficacy. In doing so, he may have had in mind the fact that his colleague, Erasmus Darwin had presented in March of the same year a description of the use of foxglove which included 6 cases he had treated. He was also careful to warn against generalising his results to all patients, because as he put it, his "cases must be considered the most hopeless and deplorable that exist; for physicians are seldom consulted in chronic diseases until the usual remedies have failed". This has relevance even today as clinicians sometimes face the problem of whether the results of randomised controlled clinical trials can be applied to their patients, if for example cases randomised to trials differ either in age, gender, ethnicity or stage of disease. Withering's skill in using foxglove will be especially appreciated by practising physicians; for even today, digoxin is unusual in the narrowness of its therapeutic range and its propensity to produce side effects due to high plasma levels or increased sensitivity, as in hypokalaemia. Withering relied on close clinical observation of his patients, in particular the pulse, severity of oedema and urine output to develop his method of dose titration and he stressed the importance of rigidly adhering to his method of dosing for any physician intending to adopt the treatment.[17]

In the 19th century, Charles Maclean (1766–1824) clearly articulated the kind of evidence that was needed to provide a reliable guide to best treatment. He advocated against relying on the advice of authority, recommending instead that claims should be confirmed or refuted by repeated experiment. As he puts it, "the verification of any result, by a repetition, under similar circumstances, of the processes by which it was originally obtained, is always best, as it is often the only evidence that can be adduced, of the accuracy of scientific conclusions: and certainly it is the only one, especially in medicine, where so much would otherwise improperly depend upon the authority of vulgar integrity" (pp. xi–x).[18] His advice was remarkably close to the concepts of evidence as advocated in our own times. However, he appears to have been less successful in practicing the methods he advocated in that much of what he reported was based on general statements and opinion.

Florence Nightingale (1820–1910) is remembered for her work as a nurse during the Crimean war. However, her impact on medical care then and later was far greater as a result of her use of reliable evidence in advocating changes. She had studied mathematics and statistics and showed how they could be used effectively for this purpose. On arriving at Scutari in 1854, she set about collecting information about the conditions she found. Her most important finding was that many more patients were dying from conditions not directly related to their injuries, but from the effects of poor nutrition, housing and sanitation within the hospital. Her use of graphics to illustrate what would otherwise appear as complex numerical data was highly effective in influencing those who read her report in government. On the basis of her records in the Crimea she published a report, Notes on Matters Affecting the Health, Efficiency, and Hospital Administration of the British Army, in 1858.[19] In this, she proposed a detailed overhaul of soldiers' living conditions and the reform of hygiene standards in hospitals. She also advocated that each hospital should maintain detailed records of all medical information related to patient care. She used diagrams and statistical data to convey her message, believing that they would "effect through the eyes what we may fail to convey to the brains of the public through their word proof ears". Nightingale's efforts had far reaching effects on hygiene and sanitary conditions in army barracks. She was also influential in reforming hospital design and management. She later became involved in the renovation of St Thomas' Hospital. Her tabulation of patient details demonstrated that most admissions originated from outside the existing catchment area and this was a key factor in deciding where to rebuild the hospital. Florence Nightingale was the first person to demonstrate convincingly the power of evidence generated by statistical methods in improving the efficiency and cost effectiveness of health care. Her methods, advocacy and impact bear remarkable resemblance to the promotion of evidence-based medicine and health economics today.

It is clear then that attempts to put medical practice on a firmer evidential base have a long history. While the amount of clinical research being undertaken and published was unprecedented towards the end of the 20th century, the fundamental nature of it was not new and awareness of the need to formalise it for optimal use in clinical practice was long established. The claim to have revealed a new paradigm for teaching and practice of medicine was unjustified and in time became something of an embarrassment for the group. Nevertheless, EBM became one of the most important movements in medicine and in time would become imbedded as a value of medical professionalism.

Summary

The term EBM was coined in the early 1990s by a group based at McMaster University as part of the launch of a new drive to shift clinical practice towards greater reliance on published evidence and randomised controlled clinical trials in particular and away from traditional reliance on experience and opinion. The EBM group advocated a new approach to medical training with a strong emphasis on literature retrieval and clinical epidemiology. The advocacy and rhetorical methods used by the group were highly successful in capturing media attention. However, it paid rather scant regard for earlier efforts to put medicine on a foundation of evidence which in fact has a long history over several centuries. The claim to have initiated a new paradigm in medical teaching and practice was not historically justified. The heavy reliance on rhetoric rather than evidence to make the case for EBM suggests an approach mostly concerned with activism and impact. In this it had considerable success both in terms of capturing the attention of the profession and the general media. It contributed to the development of a more formal and systematic approach to evaluating and interpreting clinical research. As this was the main objective of the EBM group it was successful in the medium term. It was less successful in putting forward the concept of a hierarchy of evidence which came under severe criticism for failing to acknowledge the processes by which new knowledge is acquired and for presenting an over-simplified view of clinical diagnosis and management.

References

1. Guyatt GH (1991). Evidence-based medicine (Editorial). American College of Physicians Journal Club. *Ann Int Med,* 114 (Suppl. 2), A16.
2. Evidence-Based Medicine Working Group (1992). Evidence-Based Medicine: A New Approach to Teaching the Practice of Medicine. *JAMA,* 268, 2420–2425.
3. Sackett DL, Rosenberg WM, Gray JA, Haynes RB, Richardson WS (1996). Evidence-Based Medicine: What It is and What It Isn't. *BMJ,* 312, 71–72.
4. Durack DT (1978). The Weight of Medical Knowledge. *N Eng J Med,* 298, 773–775.
5. Hitt J (2001). The Year in Ideas: A to Z; Evidence-Based Medicine. *The New York Times.* December 9.
6. Dickersin K, Straus SE, Bero LA (2007). Evidence-Based medicine: Increasing, not dictating, choice. *BMJ,* 334 (Suppl. 1), s10.
7. Benjamin Djulbegovic B, Guyatt GH, Ashcroft RE (2009). Epistemologic Inquiries in Evidence-Based Medicine. *Cancer Control,* 16, 158–168.
8. Trohler U (2000). *To Improve the Evidence of Medicine; The 18th Century British Origins of a Critical Approach.* Royal College of physicians Edinburgh.
9. Clifton F (1731). *Tabular Observations Recommended as the Plainest and Surest Way of Practising and Improving Physick.* London: Brindley.
10. Clifton F (1732). *The State of Physick, Ancient and Modern, Briefly Considered: With a Plan for the Improvement of it.* London: Printed by W Bowyer, for John Nourse without Temple-Bar.

11. Clark J (1773). Observations on Diseases in Long Voyages to Hot Countries. Available at: http://books.google.co.uk/books?id=_ZdYs8F73DMC&pg=PA111&l pg=PA111&dq=Observations+on+Diseases+in+Long+Voyages+to+Hot+Countries &source=bl&ots=pdhD7-NMz0&sig=FGsK6gWCIUs88PWknV-6Cqvum-4&hl=en&sa=X&ei=UsFzUMHRHrGZ0QWP04GoBQ&sqi=2&ved=0CB4Q6 AEwAA (Accessed on 9/10/2012)

12. Clark J (1780) Observations on Fevers Especially Those of the Continued Type, and on Scarlet Fever Attended with Ulcerated Sore Throat. Extracts of tables are available at: http://www.jameslindlibrary.org/illustrating/records/observations-on-fevers-especially-of-the-continued-type/title_pages.

13. Clark J (1792). Observations on the Diseases Which Prevail in Long Voyages to Hot Countries, Particularly on Those in the East Indies; and on the Same Diseases as they appear in Great Britain, London. Extracts of text and tables are available at: http://www.jameslindlibrary.org/illustrating/records/observations-on-the-diseases-which-prevail-in-long-voyages-to-ho/title_pages.

14. Alanson E (1782). Practical Observations on Amputation and the After Treatment. Available at: http://books.google.co.uk/books?id=kbU2Xbd7XjsC&printsec=front cover&dq=edward+alanson,+practical&source=bl&ots=tCcAZSr0eF&sig=i6gpU bbuyl6YtXSS-_uldy6vj0U&hl=en&sa=X&ei=eQl0UOjBIeTH0QWerICwDw& ved=0CDEQ6AEwAA#v=onepage&q=edward%20alanson%2C%20 practical&f=false (Accessed on 9/10/2012)

15. Cheselden W (1740). The Anatomy of the Human Body. Available at: http:// books.google.co.uk/books/about/The_Anatomy_of_the_Human_Body. html?id=yjUAAAAAQAAJ&redir_esc=y (Accessed on 9/10/2012)

16. Lind J (1753). A Treatise of Scurvy in Three Parts. Available at: detailhttp://books. google.co.uk/books?id=hytFAAAAcAAJ&printsec=frontcover&dq=james+lind,+sc urvy&source=bl&ots=S-Rhe1mHlA&sig=8WqO9pxnd4JHi1d4zfyVofwIewQ&h l=en&sa=X&ei=4I52UNCZHcmx0AXsi4HYCQ&ved=0CDEQ6AEwAA#v=on epage&q=james%20lind%2C%20scurvy&f=false (Accessed on 10/10/2012)

17. Withering W (1785). Account of the Foxglove and Some of its Medical Uses with Practical Remarks on Dropsy and Other Diseases. Available at: http://books. google.co.uk/books?id=VgIta49rzT4C&printsec=frontcover&dq=withering,+fox glove&source=bl&ots=KciZ4NFaD_&sig=Qgnrc0-fA_tknuS1yogO_ FfbXag&hl=en&sa=X&ei=Yot2UN-sGeGQ0AXgr4Eo&ved=0CDEQ6AEwAA (Accessed on 10/10/2012)

18. Maclean C (1817). Results of an Investigation, Respecting Epidemic Diseases; Including Researches in the Levant Concerning the Plague. Vol 1. Available at: http://books.google.co.uk/books?id=yS1YMhXag4kC&printsec=frontcover&d

q=charles+maclean,+1817&source=bl&ots=JWXPEFNhvK&sig=JKJcsyq7vRS
CfTyXTCHsCuwqGjI&hl=en&sa=X&ei=6sp2UIeRCJKa1AWDnIHwAg&ve
d=0CC4Q6AEwAA#v=onepage&q=charles%20maclean%2C%201817&f=
false (Accessed on 10/10/2012)

19. Aravind M, Chung KC (2009). Evidence-based medicine and hospital reform:
tracing the origins back to Florence Nightingale. *Plastic and Reconstructive
Surgery* 125, 403–409.

Chapter 2

Evidence-Based Medicine in the UK

During the 20th century, medicine advanced more rapidly than at any time in its history. In retrospect, it is not surprising that many began to question the direction that medicine was taking, its impact on society and its cost effectiveness. In the UK, two commentators were particularly significant in questioning the effectiveness of medicine and the quality of evidence on which practice was based. Archibald Cochrane's "Effectiveness and efficiency: Random Reflections on Health Services"[1] and Thomas McKeown's "The Role of Medicine: Dream, Mirage or Nemesis"[2] were perhaps the most influential books in questioning the contribution of medicine to health and in advocating a more rational evidence base for clinical practice. Although Cochrane and McKeown came from different disciplines, social medicine and public health, and their ideas differed, they are frequently cited together.[3] Cochrane is best remembered and has enjoyed something of a posthumous iconic status among advocates of evidence-based medicine (EBM) in the UK. It is perhaps ironic that Cochrane is best remembered; McKeown's analysis although it had some flaws was deeper and more convincing. Cochrane was more successful as a public health activist and rhetorician.

Thomas McKeown

Thomas McKeown (1912–1988) trained as a chemist and physiologist before studying medicine. His best known book,[2] first published in 1979 looked

19

critically at the determinants of health, particularly from the beginning of the 18th century to around 1970. His conclusion that almost all of the reduction in mortality during that period was due to better nutrition, housing and social conditions may be uncontroversial now. However, his claim that medicine played relatively little part provoked dismay among doctors and especially those in public health. Few clinicians now would dispute the importance of nutrition and living conditions on health. Public health physicians counter argued that McKeown underestimated contributions made by improved sanitation, immunisation and redistribution of resources.[4-6] In later editions of his book, McKeown went a long way to acknowledge these contributions in a thoughtful discussion (see Preface and Chapter 8, second edition).

McKeown understood and accepted that clinical medicine could have little impact on population health and mortality since it is concerned with treating people who are ill, and he valued competent medicine and humane care in helping the sick. He acknowledged that "success in prolonging life from a specific disease should be assessed in relation to those affected, rather than the general population". He repudiated those who linked his views to those of Ivan Illich who regarded the institution of medicine as a system which deprived people of the right to experience suffering. His criticism of medicine was essentially that it was having too little impact on population health and that its efforts should be refocused more on prevention, which for him involved intervening at a wide level, socially, politically, locally and globally; the important issue was the work that needed to be done by medicine, not what he called "the trade union issue" of who should do what.

McKeown combined all aspects of health care together in what he called the institution of medicine, which he saw as being charged with the care of human health in its widest context. He argued that the dominance in health care of clinical care for the sick was misguided in that it was not the best means to improve human health. Since, in his analysis medicine had contributed little to improvements in human health and that prevention is more effective than cures, he argued for increased investment in prevention if necessary at the expense of caring for the sick. However, McKeown also acknowledged that caring for the sick could never have, and is not undertaken to have, an impact on population health and that clinical care should be judged not on its ability to increase population health and longevity, but on its ability to reduce mortality in those affected. The promotion of public health and treating the sick are undertaken for related but also different reasons. Promoting health offers the possibility of longer lives, less disability and fewer sick people, but irrespective of this, the human urge to assist the ill derives from a common aspect of humanity, the expression of which is as much a necessity for human flourishing as it is for the affected individual. The society which developed an excellent system for promoting health but failed to engage with or care adequately for the frail and ill would lose an essential part of its humanity and be a miserable place for all. Indeed, McKeown acknowledged the importance of humane and Samaritan care for those who are incurable. He did not live to see the impact of modern clinical intervention on disease mortality such as in cardiovascular disease; had he done so I feel he would have had no difficulty in acknowledging it.

McKeown's main impact was two-fold; he contributed to the growing calls for greater efficiency and effectiveness in clinical care, and he charged medicine as a whole with failing to promote public health adequately. The former laid some of the ground work for advocates of EBM and reorganisation of healthcare delivery. The latter is still vigorously refuted by some public health specialists who cite the benefits of improved sanitation and claim ownership of political actions which contributed to social changes.[7] However, as mentioned above, McKeown did acknowledge the former, and he argued that the latter were attributable to economic changes. It seems to me that of McKeown's views will be uncontroversial to most clinicians today. However, the challenges in public health remain with us, a rampant global tobacco epidemic, a growing one of overweight and obesity and the, for years neglected, burden of non-communicable diseases in less developed areas of the world.

Archie Cochrane

In the UK and in many other countries, Archibald Cochrane (1909–1988) is best remembered for his work in promoting evidence-based medicine. As I have mentioned this is somewhat ironic as he came to the field late in his career and then more as an advocate than a practitioner. He is credited with promoting the use of randomised controlled trials in identifying optimal medical therapies, and in bringing the results of clinical research in an easily accessible form to clinicians; the Cochrane Collaboration which was set up to do this is named after him. Randomised controlled trials are now widely and routinely used in clinical research and accepted as essential methodology in medicine. Cochrane's name has been closely linked to this development by his many admirers around the world and as a result he is a much revered, and one might even say iconic figure today. In addition, anyone who has read his autobiography[8] will find ample evidence of courage, perseverance and generosity; he was undoubtedly a remarkable man. However, his advocacy in relation to clinical practice was far wider than simply promoting the use of randomised clinical trials. He was deeply critical of many aspects of medical practice and became part of a movement based primarily in the fields of epidemiology and public health, which sought to reform it.

The origins of Cochrane's concerns about medicine can be found very early in his career. His first contact with medical education was in Vienna, where reciprocal arrangements with Cambridge allowed him to enrol in the university. However, he found the teaching unsatisfactory and returned to London in 1934 to enter the medical school at University College Hospital. He enjoyed much of the teaching, but he tells us that he "inevitably became cynical" when he found two physicians supporting different treatments. After only two years in 1936, compelled by his passion for politics, he dropped out of medical school to serve in a field ambulance unit in Spain on the side of the democratic government. There he soon found himself triaging critically wounded soldiers. He tells us that he "hated playing God, but had to." He "tried to get medical advice as far as it was available, but the doctors were far too busy." Later, he "was called upon to give some anaesthetics (God forgive me!)". At this time too he had to triage his injured friend Julian Bell as a hopeless case, meaning that palliative care only was possible. He was clearly relieved when later in 1937, he was "ordered home to qualify".

Cochrane's political commitment and courage are much admired and rightly so. He himself was satisfied that he had made "a reasonable contribution to the anti-fascist cause, rather than merely talking about it". However, it seems obvious in retrospect that he was hopelessly unqualified both professionally and emotionally for the roles he undertook. His experiences therefore, would have been all the more harrowing. He tells us that he hated having to make life and death decisions, what he called playing God, which for someone of his inexperience and lack of knowledge would have been especially traumatic.

On returning to London he qualified in 1938 and became a house physician. He tells us he enjoyed his house job but says little of the experience he gained. However, compelled again by his antifascist sympathies he joined the army after a trip through Europe in 1939. He found himself on Crete in 1941 with the British Forces who were forced to surrender and soon after that as chief doctor in a camp holding 10,000 of his fellow prisoners of war in Salonika. It was here that he was told by a German officer that "doctors are superfluous" in response to his request for help. He appears to have been influenced by this remark which he has repeated often and at the time felt it "was probably true". However, reading his account one senses his great relief when some experienced clinicians were moved to his camp from Athens. Not long afterwards he and the camp were moved to Germany where he remained a medical officer until its liberation in 1945.

Some episodes during this time serve to illustrate his career-long attitudes towards medicine. In recounting his experience of cases of tuberculosis in the camps he recalled "cynical conversations" at medical school that "there was no real evidence apart from opinion that any treatment worked" and that in the camp he had to learn "the hard way" that surgical intervention in cases of tuberculosis carried out too early could be disastrous. For someone with so little training and experience this would indeed have been a professional and emotional challenge that few doctors would ever face. He recounts his resentment on reading a pamphlet extoling the freedom of British doctors "to do whatever they thought best for their patients" and his reaction to it; that he would gladly have sacrificed his medical freedom for some hard evidence about when to do a pneumothorax. It is clear that there would have been no randomised trials to clarify this position at the time and in retrospect I doubt that such studies would have been possible then. Cochrane clearly was a caring doctor and not infrequently to the point of exhaustion, but he also tells us that he "found caring intellectually unsatisfactory." He certainly experienced a sense of guilt for possibly shortening the lives of some of his patients due to untimely interventions and he laid the blame for this on the medical establishment for failing to provide clear evidence as to best practice and, he tells us, this would remain a theme he pursued for the remainder of his career and ultimately to his writing "Effectiveness and Efficiency".[1]

It is clear that Cochrane had a strong sense of conviction and he was committed to acting on them. However, his decision to embark on such ambitious roles on the basis of his interrupted medical studies in 1936 and his limited training in 1939 must have exacerbated the challenges and experiences he found in Spain and later in Salonika and Germany. Sir Richard Doll, who knew him, tells us in the forward to Cochrane's autobiography,[8] what distinguished Archie "from so many others of his generation was the depth of his emotional and intellectual reaction to events and his fiery independence of mind." It is clear therefore that Archie was passionate about his political views.

What is notably absent from Cochrane's recollections is a sense of his own limitations or self-criticism. His belief in the strength of his convictions may have blunted his awareness of his personal responsibility for the situations he found himself in. Even writing many decades later he shows little insight into the consequences of putting himself into the position of taking life and death decisions based on experience as a medical student. Later in Germany during WWII he found himself responsible for many thousands of fellow prisoners including a large number with tuberculosis, in which he again had limited training. It was here that he felt a sense of guilt for possibly shortening the lives of some patients as a result of untimely thoracotomies. He blames the "medical establishment" for failing to provide clear evidence for this, but appeared unaware of or discounted any possible contribution, which his own very limited clinical training and surgical skills might have contributed to his difficulties.

It is undoubtedly the case that Cochrane was poorly trained to cope with the medical challenges he faced in Spain and during WWII. That he was courageous, determined and selfless to a high degree is also undoubtedly true. He was passionate about his political views and impatient to do something about them. It is also doubtful that he would have been able to foresee the extent of the clinical problems he would face as a result of his actions. He may also have grown weary of the idea of a career in medicine as he had seen it during his training. He tells us for example that he "would never make a first rate clinician" and that he was "useless at laboratory research".

After the war, Cochrane decided on a career in public health and after training in London, and the USA he became involved in pneumoconiosis research and ran the Medical Research Council (MRC) unit based in South Wales until 1960 when it closed. He was then appointed as professor of epidemiology at Cardiff until his retirement in 1969, after which he took up the directorship of the MRC Epidemiology Unit until 1974. During this spell as professor of epidemiology he came into close contact with clinicians and medical academics and recalls his struggles in competing for financial support and teaching time on the curriculum. He also became aware through friends from his undergraduate days who had built careers in the MRC and the Department of Health and Social Security (DHSS) that health services research was a developing priority for the latter. At this time, the DHSS was being increasingly pressed by the Treasury over rising healthcare costs and inflation associated with new treatments and new hospitals.[9] He decided to steer his new unit in this direction and successfully approached contacts at the MRC for financial support for this. With guidance from contacts at the DHSS, he began to direct his efforts towards evaluating the effectiveness of therapies which had been developed in the National Health Service (NHS). This work brought him increasingly into contact with like-minded individuals such as Thomas McKeown and Alan Williams (who had been an economic advisor to the treasury, liaising between it and the DHSS), as well as organisations promoting health services research, the MRC, the DHSS and The Nuffield Trust. It was the Nuffield Trust at the instigation (Cochrane tells us) of the DHSS which invited and sponsored his writing "Effectiveness and Efficiency; Random Reflections on Health Services". The book was largely a rhetorical piece and Archie's opinions would have been well known to those involved in sponsoring him; it can be seen therefore as an effort to further the interests of health services research instigated from the DHSS, operating behind the scenes.[10]

Cochrane's book is a remarkable accomplishment in many ways. It is eminently engaging, readable, amusing and is written with what appears to be an almost boyish sense of fun. It heralded and predicted important changes that have occurred in medicine in the past century. Its success in convincing so many probably owes as much to the disarming quality of Cochrane's anecdotes and style as to the quality of the evidence he presented. He rarely allows a serious point to stand alone without some little jest to lighten the impact on his audience. The result is more a work of advocacy (some might say agitprop) than of reasoned argument. The approach has served well in publicising the case for greater scrutiny of the cost effectiveness of medicine, but it may also have served to distract from the seriousness of his intent and from rigorous critique of his views. That Cochrane's approach was deeply affecting is demonstrated by many who have subsequently reported "life changing experiences" having met him or read his book.[9] Most, it must be said, were already committed to the concepts of health economics or were drawn to the field of epidemiology; I have found it much more difficult to find detailed comments from career-committed clinicians. For example, his lecture in 1978 sponsored by the Office of Health Economics,[11] in which he reiterated many of his views, was part of a symposium which gave no serious opportunity to reflect on their potential impact on the practice of clinical medicine. Furthermore, the 25th anniversary of Archie's lecture was celebrated with a new book, "Non-random reflections on health services research"[12] which extoled Cochrane's views and the advances made in health services research, but once again I struggled to find any clinicians among the contributors or indeed among reviewers of it.

Cochrane made much about clinicians objecting to randomised controlled trials, whom he regularly accused of "playing God" or of suffering from the "God complex", phrases which appear repeatedly in his book.[1] In a paper entitled "Archie Cochrane, An Internal Challenge to Physicians' Autonomy?"[13] again written by an epidemiologist, the only reference to physicians autonomy comes from a discussion among sociologists. In fact there seems to be remarkably little written by practicing clinicians about Cochrane, the movement he represented or what its implications were for medicine. This seems to me regrettable because although his main message about cost effectiveness was a good one, Cochrane had other views about medicine that had nothing to do with autonomy and which in some respects were highly damaging for medicine. I suspect that many agreed with his central message and overlooked his tendency to stereotype, oversimplify and exaggerate; others may have regarded his criticism as amusing satire and not in need of comment.

What then were Archie's views about medicine? His main thrust was to insist on the introduction of systems to determine the efficacy of all treatments available in the NHS and their effectiveness for which randomised controlled trials would be used. He set out his vision of measuring the cost effectiveness of the NHS with a list of inputs and outputs. The inputs included, for example all medical and other research "which is of use to the NHS in carrying out its objectives". The NHS, he argued, "cannot claim any credit for this external input. It can only be judged by the use that is made of it." He then went on to give a list of some of these inputs such as penicillin, anti-tuberculous drugs, anti-hypertensives, steroids, anti-depressants, which he reminded us had never been greater in any comparable period in history. This he claimed raised the level of what might be expected of the NHS, given "the magnificent quality of this external input". But this is of course, a profoundly misguided view of the contributions which the NHS and clinical as well as many other branches of medicine made to medical science. Indeed, none of the advances he mentioned could have been possible without multiple contributions from researchers based in the NHS at many levels. For example, understanding the nature of diseases is an essential prerequisite to developing new treatments for them and new treatments must be evaluated in a clinical context, all of which requires support of health services. Cochrane's narrow conception of cost benefit analysis is well illustrated by his approach to coronary care units (CCU).

One of the most engaging parts of Cochrane book was his discussion of his involvement in the introduction of these new units. Here he revels in combative language; "the battle for coronary care is just beginning" (p. 51).[1] He seems to have had a particular antipathy for cardiologists whom he described as "the Tuscany set" and being infected with a heavy dose of the "God complex". He became aware of concerns about the potential costs of CCUs from contacts in the DHSS and he set about carrying out a study of their cost effectiveness. He describes objections from cardiologists about difficulties which they foresaw in randomising acutely ill patients with myocardial infarction and he regales his readers with some amusing anecdotes of scoring over his bêtes noires. In the event, the trial went ahead[14] and showed no difference in mortality between patients randomly allocated to home versus hospital treatment. This was hailed by Cochrane as a success and of course it was in some ways, but for many clinicians the randomisation rate achieved of just 28% (63% were electively admitted to hospital) limited its usefulness. In a follow-up report of an extension to the study[15] this fell even further to just 23% of all patients seen. The trial also showed that hypotension was a significant predictor of risk for increased mortality and that GPs may have been aware of this in that they electively admitted more patients with hypotension. There was also a worrying higher incidence of hypotension among patients randomised to hospital treatment. These findings in fact confirm the cardiologists concerns that difficulties in randomisation[16,17] would very likely be encountered during a trial and limit its usefulness. To a determined health economist seeking a yes or no answer to a simple question this might have seemed like intransigence, but they were perfectly correct in pointing them out and would have been irresponsible had they not done so. For a trial which has little prospect of providing useful information, challenging questions about its own ethics and cost effectiveness also arise. This episode illustrates well Cochrane's vision for the future of clinical medicine. His view of cost benefit analysis, focussed exclusively on mortality outcomes, important as this is, effectively ignored and discounted contributions that CCUs were making to advance this field of medicine; advances which in time became a major contributor to reducing coronary heart disease mortality.

This conception of medical science as an external input to the NHS and clinical medicine was a major distortion implicit in Cochrane's views about health care. His belief that the NHS could claim no credit for any developments in medical science meant that research undertaken by clinicians and others working in the NHS or funded by it would also have made no contribution to it. The fallacy of this is also well exemplified by the only important randomised clinical trial with which Cochrane was ever associated.[18] This was the report of one of the earliest studies of the efficacy of aspirin in preventing mortality from myocardial infarction. Like all clinical trials, its ethical justification required that there was a reasonable expectation that patients could gain some benefit from it and that there was a sound scientific basis for subjecting patients to the inconvenience and risks involved. The rational basis for the hypothesis tested in that study was (a) evidence that aspirin was capable of inhibiting thrombosis by its recently discovered anti-platelet action and (b) the also recent confirmation that myocardial infarction was caused by coronary thrombosis. One of the references cited in support of (a) was a publication from researchers based at his own institution and a nearby NHS hospital.[19] The work of these researchers included clinical research in patients with myocardial infarction[20] and it is inconceivable that this could have been done without their experience in clinical medicine and support from the NHS. The paper cited no references in relation to (b). Thrombosis had been much discussed in relation to myocardial infarction for many years at this time. However, controversy remained about whether it was causal or a post-mortem occurrence.[21,22] Proof that intracoronary thrombosis was the primary cause of acute myocardial infarction had in fact only recently been emerging based on careful documentation of the natural history of the acute event together with detailed pathological studies (for review see Ref. 23). The work that led to this was made possible by clinicians and pathologists[24] deeply involved in practice and the close observation of patients made possible by the introduction of CCUs and would not have been possible without the input and the support of the NHS. This of course is also true of clinical services in other countries however, they may be organised.

This denial of the contribution of others to science is not merely a lack of generosity, it more importantly distorts understanding of how science works and negates its value. For anyone familiar with the workings of the NHS I am sure its contribution to medical science both direct and indirect, would have been obvious. Cochrane however derided it, describing research carried out in the NHS as "phenomenological and pseudo-research", as a waste of resources creating inefficiency. He was especially harsh about pathology which he described as "a minor function", and an anachronism that would be "replaced by medical scientists who will measure the effectiveness and efficiency of therapy and in conjunction with social scientists assess the adequacy of community care". These views were not "random reflections"; they were in fact central to his vision of the future. They allowed Cochrane, for example, to suggest that measures of cost effectiveness of health care systems such as CCU's could be carried out ignoring any contribution they make to medical advances and thereby to undermine the value of clinical science. They also served to bolster his argument that measures of healthcare cost effectiveness and efficiency (what he called applied research) were cheaper than hypothesis driven science (what he called phenomenological research) and should replace it. He anticipated that as funding for "phenomenological research was reduced physicians will interest themselves in applied research".

Cochrane was wrong about CCUs. They flourished and made major contributions to understanding coronary heart disease and its treatment. At the time of writing Efficacy and Efficiency,[1] he cited standardised mortality rates for ischaemic heart disease, which at the time were still rising, to illustrate inefficiencies in medicine. However, they would soon begin to decline and become one of the most successful reversals of medical prognosis for a non-communicable disease. He did not have the opportunity to see this and to contribute to analysing the factors responsible for it, namely the advances in treatment and prevention and the discoveries in medical science which led to them.[25] He was wrong in his portrayal of doctors in general as being opposed to the introduction of randomised controlled clinical trials. Ironically, one of the most striking contributions of CCUs was in facilitating some of the most ambitious clinical trials done to evaluate and compare treatments for patients with acute myocardial infarction. In his autobiography,[8] Cochrane tells us that he always responded to questions about home versus hospital care for myocardial infarction by insisting he would choose home care. He describes how consideration of this became a personal reality when he had what he self-diagnosed as a "coronary". However, this diagnosis may also reflect a life-long over confidence in his clinical abilities. He described an episode in the 1980s when he suddenly felt very ill with vague abdominal pains and retching. He continued to be unwell over the next two days and consulted his GP who found his blood pressure reduced and suggested an ECG. This showed "reversed T waves in one lead" and he "realised I had had a coronary". However, these clinical features are not typical of myocardial infarction and they certainly would not have satisfied the diagnostic criteria set out in the clinical trial he cited so frequently.[14]

In advocating for investment in health economics and what would be called health related research, Cochrane cited what he saw as several other inefficiencies in healthcare. He argued for example that sick leave from work was a "real output of the NHS as it is time off certified by doctors under contract to the NHS". In other words, if a worker suffered a broken arm due to an accident at work and had time off work, this counted as an NHS output if it was supported by a GP's signature. He then went on to show that work days lost due to sick leave were greater than to industrial action and concluded that "the NHS was a disaster for the economy". He then explained how he had organised malingering among prisoners of war camps in Germany to give them some respite. He did not directly accuse GPs of doing so, but again the anecdote illustrates his rhetorical skill in inviting the reader to think that they may have be doing so without providing any evidence for it. He also had strong views on population control. He recommended abortion because it was "less demanding on the resources of the NHS than childbirth and because he did not believe that making contraception or vasectomy available would be effective". He expressed sympathy for gynaecologists because as he put it "I can appreciate that the operation of abortion is often unpleasant and that some of the clients do not appear as particularly worthy citizens". He felt that "refusal to abort" should be a registered medical condition.

In calling for improvements in efficiency and effectiveness in healthcare, Cochrane was stating the obvious. Who would argue against it? He was also pushing against an open door in that rising healthcare costs was causing alarm in governments. This may also explain his remarkable foresight in predicting the rise of qualitative research, what he called applied research or health related research, as funding for original clinical science was withdrawn over succeeding decades.[26,27] He made the case for this using powerful rhetoric, which included some deeply flawed and sometimes odious views. However, his account of these events suggests that he was laying the ground work for policies which had already evolved and had political weight. His task therefore may not have been to develop well-reasoned arguments in support, but rather one of activism to help implement them and in this of course he was highly successful.

Randomised controlled trials were to be the tools of raising efficiency and effectiveness in medicine, as they were for the implementation of EBM (discussed in Chapter 1). Their introduction as a means to establish optimal therapies in medicine was one of the most important developments in medicine in the 20th century. This was in fact well recognised and embraced within mainstream medicine; and is now recognised as essential elements in 21st century medical professionalism.[28] Indeed, their rapid take up generally proved so great that in just a few years Cochrane was again critical of medicine; "It is surely a great criticism of our profession that we have not organised a critical summary, by speciality or subspecialty, adapted periodically, of all relevant randomised controlled trials."[11] This heralded the creation of a new enterprise named after Cochrane aimed at evaluating published trials and packaging reviews for health workers. These reviews which are widely admired and valued are undertaken by groups of workers all over the world with the enthusiastic involvement of clinicians. They are, however, reviews of past work, derivative in nature and unoriginal in terms of scientific enquiry. This represents exactly the kind of health related research which Cochrane advocated so strongly and predicted would emerge as funding for original research was withdrawn. Not surprisingly, it also coincided with the decline in academic medicine and clinical discovery and the failure to translate new discoveries in biology into clinical practice.[29] Its emphasis, as implicit in all qualitative research, is to make the best use of what we have rather than seeking to make new discoveries. A couple of examples illustrate this well. We have endless publications and guidelines about how to best use the prostate specific antigen test for prostate cancer and warnings about its inappropriate use. On the other hand, it is rare to find the question asked, why are we still relying on such an outdated and unreliable test and why have we not invested in research adequately to discover a better one? And then we have repeated warnings about the dangers of antibiotic resistance; the problem is presented as one of their improper use and hygiene failure. However, important both of these measures are, given the inevitability that bacteria will develop resistance to all our present drugs in due course, it is misguided not to invest adequately in research to discover new ones. Both examples illustrate the present emphasis of the qualitative research approach at the expense of original science, as Cochrane advocated, and how this has eroded our ability to make new discoveries. He may have been right to advocate for improved efficiency in healthcare; his view that this should be at the expense of degrading our capacity for original medical science was misguided and has contributed to its decline in recent decades.

Summary

Thomas McKeown and Archie Cochrane are most frequently associated with the origins of EBM in the UK. McKeown, an academic sociologist was motivated by his analysis of the determinants of human health. His conclusion that social and economic factors were most important led him to argue for the redirection of resources towards them if necessary at the expense of direct health care, for more reliance on prevention and less on cure. He encountered opposition from some in public health for failure to acknowledge contribution in sanitation and political action to promote changes in social conditions. McKeown did acknowledge these, and he also recognised the importance of caring for the sick including Samaritan and palliative.

Archie Cochrane was a leading voice in calling for improved efficiency in health care delivery. He appears to have been motivated by a lifelong dystopian view of medicine, having found his initial contact in Vienna "unsatisfactory", tending towards "cynicism" as a medical student and blaming the "medical establishment" for many of the difficulties he experienced in caring for prisoners of war. He was antipathetic towards clinical medicine and medical science. He regarded research within the health service as wasteful "phenomenology" and argued for its replacement with applied "health related research". This would take the form of health economics and systematic reviews of clinical trials by specialty. The latter led to a new enterprise named after him with contributors from all over the world, discussed in Chapter 3. In this he was highly successful as applied qualitative research has expanded rapidly in the past two decades, just as he predicted it would as investment in original science was withdrawn.

This expansion of qualitative research coincided with the decline in academic medicine. Cochrane saw no dangers in this as he regarded it as wasteful. Therefore he could not have foreseen the decline in clinical discovery and the failure to translate new discoveries in biology into clinical practice that would follow. He is a much admired, even revered figure, which may explain why these negative aspects of his legacy have been overlooked and are now emerging as a serious impediment to medical progress.

References

1. Cochrane A (1972). Effectiveness and Efficiency: Random Reflections on Health Services. London, Nuffield Provincial Trust p. xiii–xv.
2. McKeown (1979). The Role of Medicine: Dream, Mirage or Nemesis. London, Nuffield Provincial Trust and Blackwell, Oxford.
3. Alvarez-Dardet, Ruiz C, Thomas McKeown MT, Cochrane A (1993). A Journey through the Diffusion of Ideas. *BMJ*, 306, 1252–1255.
4. Szretzer S (1988). The Importance of Social Intervention in Britain's Mortality Decline c1850–1914: A Re-interpretation of the Role of Public Health. *Social History of Medicine*, 1, 1–37.
5. Cosgrave J (2002). The McKeown Thesis: A Historical Controversy and its Enduring Influence. *Am J Pub Health*, 92, 725–732.
6. Szretzer S (2002). Rethinking McKeown: The Relationship between Public Health and Social Change. *Am J Pub Health*, 92, 722–725.
7. Szretzer S (2003). Rethinking McKeown. *Am J Pub Health*, 93, 1032–1033.
8. Cochrane AL, Blythe M (2009) One Man's Medicine. Cardiff University Publication.
9. Williams A (1997). All Cost Effectiveness Treatments should be free ... or, how Archie Coachrane Changed my Life! *J Epid and Pub Health*, 51, 116–120.

10. Sally Sheard, Liam Donaldson (2006). The Nation's Doctor, The role of the Chief Medical Officer 1855–1998, Chapter 6. Oxford, Seattle: Radcliffe Publishing.

11. Cochrane AL (1931–1971). A Critical Review with Particular Reference to the Medical Profession. *In*: Medicines for the year 2000. London: Office of Health Economics, pp. 2–12.

12. Non-random reflections on health services research, On the 25th Anniversary of Archie Cochrane's Effectiveness and Efficiency. (Ed). A Maynard and I Chalmers. London: BMJ Publishing group.

13. Hill GB (2000). Archie Cochrane and his Legacy, an Internal Challenge to Physicians' Autonomy? *J Clin Epid*, 53, 1190–1192.

14. Mather HG, Pearson NG, Read KLQ, Shaw DB, Steed GR, Thorne MG, Jones S, Guerrier CJ, Eraut CD, Mchugh PM, Chowdhury NR, Jafary MH, Wallace TJ (1971). Acute Myocardial Infarction: Home and Hospital Treatment. *BMJ*, 3, 334–338.

15. Mather HG, Morgan DC, Pearson NG, Thorne MG, Lawrence CJ, Riley IS (1976). Myocardial Infarction: A Comparison between Home and Hospital Care for Patients. *BMJ*, 1, 925–926.

16. Oliver MF, Julian DG, Donald KW (1967). Problems in Evaluating Coronary Care Units. Their Responsibilities and their Relation to the Community. *Am J Cardiol*, 20, 465–474.

17. Julian DG (2001). The Evolution of the Coronary Care Unit. *Cardiovasc Res*, 51, 621–624.

18. Elwood PC, Cochrane AL, Burr ML, Sweetnam PM, Williams G, Welsby E, Hughes SJ, Renton R (1974). A Randomized Controlled Trial of Acetyl Salicylic Acid in the Secondary Prevention of Mortality from Myocardial Infarction. *BMJ*, 1(5995), 436–440.

19. Davies DTP, Hughes A, Tonks RS (1968). *Archiv Fur Experimentelle Pathologie und Pharmakologie*, 259, 163.

20. Hughes A, Tonks RS (1966). Magnesium, Adenosine Diphosphate and Blood Platelets. *Nature* 210, 106–107.

21. Baroldi G (1965). Acute Coronary Occlusion as a Cause of Myocardial Infarct and Sudden Coronary Death. *Am J Cardiol*, 16, 859.

22. Roberts WC, Buja LM (1972). The Frequency and Significance of Coronary Arterial Thrombi and Other Observations in Fatal Acute Myocardial Infarction. *Am J Med*, 52, 425.

23. Davies MJ, Woolf N, Robertson WB (1976). Pathology of Acute Myocardial Infarction with Particular Reference to Occlusive Coronary Thrombi. *Br Heart J*, 38, 659–664.

24. Armstrong A, Duncan B, Oliver MF (1972). Natural History of Acute Coronary Heart Attacks. *Br Heart J*, 34, 67–80.

25. Smolina K, Wright FL, Rayner M, Goldacre MJ (2012). Determinants of the Decline in Mortality from Acute Myocardial Infarction in England between 2002 and 2010: Linked National Database Study. *BMJ*, 344.

26. Clinical Academic Medicine in Jeopardy. Academy of Medical Sciences. Available at: http://www.google.co.uk/url?sa=t&rct=j&q=&esrc=s&frm=1&sour ce=web&cd=1&ved=0CC4QFjAA&url=http%3A%2F%2Fwww.acmedsci. ac.uk%2Fdownload.php%3Ffile%3D%2Fimages%2Fpublication%2Fpclin aca.pdf&ei=wJK0UIbnM4ST0QXahYHQBw&usg=AFQjCNFOiARHetDA1 poPUBxPNMiNjlT0Wg (Accessed on 26/11/2012).

27. Sheridan DJ (2006). Reversing the Decline of Academic Medicine in Europe. *Lancet*, 367, 1698–1701.

28. Medical professionalism in the new millennium (2002). A physicians' Charter. *Lancet*, 359, 520–522.

29. Sheridan DJ (2013). *Medical Science in the 21st Century; Sunset or New dawn.* London: Imperial College Press.

Chapter 3

The Cochrane Collaboration

The largest and most important development from the evidence-based medicine (EBM) movement has been the Cochrane Collaboration. The idea is said to have come from a comment in an assay by Archie Cochrane published in 1979 by the UK Office of Health Economics.[1] Cochrane had originally argued in his 1972 monograph that randomised controlled trials would be the tools for improving efficiency in healthcare.[2] His original rhetoric that the medical profession was strongly opposed to their introduction proved to be incorrect and so much so that by 1979 his criticism changed to "It is surely a great criticism of our profession that we have not organised a critical summary, by speciality or subspecialty, adapted periodically, of all relevant randomised controlled trials". The collaboration developed out of discussions between members of the EBM movement from the UK and McMaster University and received its initial funding from the UK Department of Health (DH) and the Nuffield Trust. The first Cochrane Centre opened in 1992 in Oxford primarily concerned with producing systematic reviews of the literature related to pregnancy and childhood health, the specialism of its founder Iain Chalmers.

The concept of a wider collaboration was put forward by Chalmers in 1993.[3] By then, four centres had been established in the UK, Canada, Sweden and the USA and it was proposed to extend the collaboration both geographically, and to cover health care more widely. The structure had been developed and was based on recruiting groups of volunteers to work in specific areas based on their expertise. Review groups were coordinated by an editorial team, which also produced an edited version of reviews. These were then deposited in a database of systematic reviews. The initial review group dealing with pregnancy and childbirth had 30 reviewers committed to writing and maintaining 500–600 reviews of randomised controlled trials, and to incorporating 200–300 new trials, each year. Funding for the work of volunteers was raised by the volunteers themselves and the editorial team and central administration was supported by the UK DH.

In the same year, preparation of a handbook to standardise the preparation of systematic reviews began and was published in 1994. The concept of systematic reviews proved highly popular to governments and funders of health care, and so expansion occurred rapidly during the succeeding years. New review groups were formed to cover a wide range of medical treatments and with a global distribution. In 1995, a database of systematic reviews was launched by the UK DH, and a new steering group was elected. A new library as a quarterly publication on CD-ROM was opened in 1996 and the database of systematic reviews was made available on the WEB in the same year. In 2003, a Chief Executive Officer was appointed and an agreement was signed with a major publisher. The collaboration met annually to review its progress and strategy, 2012 marking its 20th anniversary. For a more detailed history of the collaboration, see Ref. 4.

Annual publication of new reviews was 402 in 2009, 449 in 2010 and in 416 in 2011; updated reviews for the same period were 479, 524 and 468 respectively.[5] The total number of published reviews has increased as the collaboration has expanded from 2,000 in 2004 to 4,713 by 2011.[5] Originally planned to be updated every two years, the percentage for which this was achieved was around one-third, declining from 39.8% in 2009 to 35.8% in 2012.[5] Evidence of the usefulness and popularity of reviews can be derived from their bibliometrics. In 2010, full text downloads from the Cochrane library were 3,956,567. The 5 most frequently downloaded reviews accounted for 43,314 of these and related to health interventions to treat or prevent falls (2), obesity (2) and leg ulcers (1).[6] The impact factor of the Cochrane library, a measure of how frequently it is used by other researchers in comparison with other research publications, increased steadily from 4.654 in 2007 to 5.182 in 2008, 5.653 in 2009 and 6.186 in 2010, which placed it 10th highest in that year.[6]

The preparation of systematic reviews is undertaken by volunteer contributors around the world. The total number amounted to over 40,000 in 2013.[7] In 2009, these worked in 53 review groups based in 29 centres and branches around the world, 12 in Europe, 2 in the USA, 4 in South America, 2 in Africa, 2 in China and 1 in Canada, Australia, New Zealand, India, Thailand, Singapore and Bahrain.[8] Authors from low and middle income countries accounted for 21.3% in 2009, 18.4% in 2010 and 21.5% in 2011.[5]

Funding

Initial funding for the collaboration was provided by the UK DH and the Nuffield Trust. Both have a long interest in health care economics. Cochrane's original lecture and monograph[2] were sponsored by the Nuffield Trust and, as Cochrane tells us in his autobiography, at the instigation of the DH. Development of the Cochrane Library has provided a source of regular funding for the core activities of the collaboration. The total income received by the collaboration was around £20 million in 2009–2010. Approximately, 90% of this was raised by review groups locally to fund their research and preparation of reviews. The sources of group's funding in 2009 were predominantly (79%) government or trans-government grants with charities providing around 8%, and sales from the Cochrane library 6%.[8] Core funding, which support the central functions of the collaboration comes mainly from the proceeds of the Cochrane library, which accounted for 6% of the total income in 2009.[8] A fundamental element of the collaboration's mission is avoidance of bias in its reviews. For this reason, it does not accept support or sponsorship from the pharmaceutical industry or for-profit industries that provide healthcare services. Government departments, not for profit insurance companies and health management organisations that may have an interest in review outcomes are not prohibited.

These figures represent formal funding arrangements. However, the collaboration is heavily built around contributing volunteers. There is no suggestion that this is provided in free time and the support of host institutions is readily acknowledged. In a sense therefore volunteers are offering time paid for by their employers and with their permission, which in most cases is likely to be either health services or academic institutions. The value in kind of this effort is difficult to assess. Some indication may be gleaned from the suggestion by the current CEO that it would take in the region of $1 billion per annum to set up now using a standard commercial model and to purchase the outputs of the collaboration now would cost £100 billion.[6] The collaboration is certainly a major enterprise with most of the work being done by unpaid contributors, who are more often researchers than clinicians. A hidden cost in all of this is the work, both research and clinical, which is relegated to accommodate support for the collaboration. That this redirection of effort should occur was always part of Cochrane's vision. He argued that clinical research carried out in the health service, what he called phenomenology, made no contribution to medical progress, was wasteful and should be replaced by applied research of the kind done by the collaboration (pp. 12, 44, 81, 83).[2] The EBM movement and the collaboration named after him can therefore be seen as a major effort to enact Cochrane's vision and that of his backers. The value of the collaboration's work is beyond question; however, no attempt has been made to measure its indirect costs. Redirecting investment away from clinical science has resulted in the decline of academic medicine, medical discoveries and innovation. In addition, the redirection of the effort of many thousands of epidemiologists and public health researchers has limited efforts to tackle serious failures in public health, the epidemics of overweight and obesity and misuse of tobacco and alcohol.

There is currently a broad consensus that systematic reviews are a valuable and important contribution to communicating advances in medicine. There is also convincing evidence that up to date cumulative meta analyses are superior to traditional reviews, and textbooks for rapid dissemination of new research findings.[9] Systematic reviews provide clinicians with rapid up to date information to help guide best practice. Cochrane reviews are also intended to guide policy making in deciding health priorities, in relation to health needs and available resources.[3] The fact that so much of its funding comes from health providing organisations attests to its usefulness. Thus, the strength of the collaboration is its ability to provide rapid summations of research to inform clinical decisions and health policy formulation. Depending on the timeliness of its reviews and updates of them, it has the capacity to do this more accurately and quickly than was available previously.

Future Challenges

As experience has grown, new challenges and weaknesses in the collaboration have also emerged mainly, it must be said, from its collaborators and supporters. Almost inevitably the question arises as to what areas of medicine does it cover and what subjects does it provide reviews for? It is generally acknowledged that even with 5,000 current reviews published to date, coverage is patchy.[10] Some reviews reflect the interests of authors but may be too diffuse or too focused to be of use to clinicians, or they may wastefully overlap with similar reviews by other groups.[7] To some extent, this is not surprising since topics are often selected by volunteer groups reflecting their personal interests. This is a challenge recognised by the collaboration and mechanisms to counter it have been proposed, including publishing overviews of systematic reviews,[11] developing methods for identifying high priority topics[12,13] being more aligned with the needs of stake holder organisations and developing policies to manage the selection of topics to register.[7] Such changes would be significant for the collaboration. It has developed as a bottom-up organisation attracting thousands of highly committed volunteers, most of whom are researchers with individual interests. Moving to a more directed top-down approach would be a major change of tack. One founder of the collaboration likened "Cochranites" to the Jesuits as passionate believers in the mission, who often "work for free" and are "signed up for life". Whether they would be as inclined to be as obedient to a directed top-down approach as an order of monks is difficult to predict. Researchers, at least those engaged in original science are generally independently minded. Cochrane himself certainly believed in a directed approach. He saw a clear distinction between the applied research which the collaboration does and original science, the former based on pre-ordained hypotheses, examined using readymade protocols in contrast to the original questions and methods of investigative science (p. 80).[2]

How successful the collaboration will be in developing a more directed approach to topic selection as Cochrane envisaged remains to be seen. There seems little doubt that the extent of the challenge it represents to the collaboration was recognised early on. One of its principal founders, Iain Chalmers, later developed the James Lind Alliance, named after James Lind (1716–1794) famous for his original discoveries for treating scurvy, to identify and set priority research questions. Funded again by the UK DH, its goal is to identify priority questions in healthcare by consensus among its many affiliated groups and organisations.[14] The hope is that this will help to manage the direction of science in general as well as the selection of areas for systematic reviews by the collaboration.

Discussion of topic selection within the collaboration is confined within the limits of its present mission, which mainly covers therapeutic interventions. Extension to include even diagnostic methods is resisted. Its standard defence against mission creep today is its finite resources. However, this would not have been the case at the time of its creation. The focus on treatments was justified by the need to improve the uptake of optimal therapy. But there are many other areas of healthcare with similar or even greater needs. For example, failures in public health due to overweight and obesity, the missuse of tobacco and alcohol and inequality are some of our greatest health challenges today. The collaboration's unwillingness to include policy interventions to tackle these in its mission is to say the least disturbing and even more so, since many of its supporters and collaborators are based in the fields of epidemiology and public health.

Arguably the greatest area of need for evidence-based practice in medicine today is in health policy. Initiatives related to delivery of care are almost always announced in an evidence vacuum. This frequently results in confusion and controversy[15] as exemplified in the UK by the introduction of the new National Health Service (NHS) helpline, "NHS 111"[16] and the Health and Social Care Act.[17] The Cochrane Collaboration does not address the evidence base for health policy because its selective mission excludes it. But even if it were included, it is highly unlikely that the collaboration would be able to contribute significantly to it. This is due to a fundamental weakness of all comparative research. Its objective is to review what has already been studied rather than to investigate anything new; and so if there is a paucity of primary research it can only be silent. Thus, the collaboration produces a large volume of health related research, much of which is useful. However, the sheer volume of its output and its impact on the health agenda, which will need to increase further if it is to meet its objectives, coupled with its selective mission contribute to masking large gaps where primary research is desperately needed to guide health policy more effectively. In other words, research is important not just for what it covers but for what it does not. Thus, in relation to health policy we have the paradox that policy initiatives related to delivery of care are introduced on a background of little evidence or follow-up research, whereas policy changes aimed at protecting public health, such as plain tobacco packaging,[18] are required to be supported by the highest levels of evidence before implementation.

The collaboration takes great care to avoid accepting funds or support from industries linked to health care, in order to avoid potential conflicts of interest. But that still leaves the question as to whether the sources of its initial funding influenced its choice of direction and mission at the outset. To a large degree the collaboration has been funded by providers of health care and some of those have been responsible for the introduction of multiple reforms, many of which have never been subject to any form of review or assessment. It begs the question; would the collaboration have been so successful in securing this funding if it had been committed to evaluating the impact of such reforms? Conflicts of interest should be avoided, not only when they threaten immediate goals, but also when they may influence overall strategy and mission. The collaboration loses no opportunity to remind us that it avoids conflicts of interest in relation to the reviews it sponsors, however, there could well be potential for conflict between the selective nature of its mission in health care and its main sources of income.

Mission Creep

It is not surprising that an organisation which has grown so rapidly should encounter challenges and problems along the way. It is to its credit that the collaboration not only recognises this, but actively searches for them at its annual gatherings. The issue of mission creep is a recurring one.[7,10] For the time being it seems likely the collaboration will stick to its original statement, but criticism of this position will continue since all aspects of health care need to be evidence based. Objections to expanding its role are principally a lack of resources and the fact that it has much to do simply to meet its current objectives.

Efficiency

Publication and maintenance of 5,000 systematic reviews is a substantial achievement. However, this has been achieved while the collaboration has received approximately £150 million, equivalent to £30,000 per review. In addition, it has the service of 40,000 volunteers who undertake most of this work without payment. Furthermore, reviews are only as valuable as they are kept up to date and as of 2012 only 35% satisfied the collaborations own definition for this requirement.[5] Time is also an issue; at present, it takes on average 30 months to produce a review. Some critics already see this as evidence that the present system is unsustainable in the long term.[19] Collaboration insiders recognise the need to develop new strategies to improve efficiency. Approaches under consideration include developing faster literature search techniques, prioritising reviews and updates of them[20] and developing automated review processes.[21] It seems likely that further resources would be needed to increase the frequency of review updates and particularly so as the accumulating number of reviews increases over time. Cutting back on the number of review groups has been suggested as one means to improve efficiency and free up resources.[7] However, it is unclear whether this can be achieved without undermining the enthusiasm of its volunteers on which the entire system depends.

The collaboration sets high standards for its reviews; it has 80 standards for the conduct of reviews and 108 for reporting reviews.[22] However, most reviews fail to meet all of these standards, resulting in varying quality.[5] Once again, the collaboration is aware of this and a string of improvements have been proposed.[7] The real challenge will be whether greater uniformity of its output can be achieved without fundamentally altering the bottom-up nature of the collaboration. Despite these challenges, it offers the best system for preparing and publishing systematic reviews available at present. But it is not without competition. Already independent academic units provide large numbers of important and valuable meta-analyses and I suspect this will increase, as the commercial potential of accumulating portfolios of reviews becomes more widely appreciated. The value of the collaboration's archive is already substantial. It generated an income of around £1.8 million in 2009 and £2.4 million in 2010 and this can only increase with the size and range of its portfolio.[8] Its asset value is more difficult to assess, but the current CEO has estimated that it would be around £100 billion to purchase outright.[6] In the economic environment we live in, it is inconceivable that such a lucrative market will be left to the exclusive use of just one provider. Furthermore, the collaboration has established a platform for influencing clinical management on the basis of a high level of integrity, and has the potential to have a major impact on the market of health products. Again it seems unimaginable that others will not try to muscle in on such an enterprise.

Already, alternative and less costly approaches to reviews are being considered. For example a random sample of Cochrane reviews compared with the largest and best of the randomised controlled clinical trials showed agreement in 81% of cases.[23] An important standard for Cochrane reviews is the literature search for possible trials to include in their analysis, based on the Cochrane Controlled Trials Register, Medline and Ambase. The extensive nature of this adds to the work and cost of producing reviews. A simpler search for adding trials to update reviews would reduce the work involved, but might also reduce their accuracy. Comparison of the McMaster Premium Literature Service (PLUS) with the standard Cochrane approach showed similar results, but PLUS identified only 23% of the trials included in the Cochrane approach, suggesting that some simplification may be achievable without loss of accuracy.[24] A further approach to simplification has been studied, by comparing meta-analyses based on trials in a selected set of specialist and general journals with Cochrane systematic reviews,[25] and found that almost all of the findings were replicated. It seems clear that the market for systematic reviews and meta-analyses will continue to evolve. It is also likely that other players will emerge over time. The Cochrane Collaboration's experience and reputation will also keep it at the forefront of the field.

Science or Market Research?

The history of the Cochrane Collaboration originates in the EBM movement. Launched on a similar wave of rhetoric[3] harking back to the views of its icon Archie Cochrane,[1] and the McMaster group,[26] it emerged as an obvious "must-have" and grew rapidly with support from health provider organisations. A question which seems to have attracted little discussion is how should its work be categorised? It generally falls under the heading of "health related research", but this conveys little meaning. Is it Science? Is it market research? Is it a kind of "best-buy" research for medicines? Or is it research to assist regulation of new health interventions? For some it may be sufficient that it provides valuable and useful resources.

The issue is important for two reasons. First, the nature of the work the Cochrane Collaboration does has a bearing on how it is funded and second, the future benefits we can and cannot expect from its work depend on the kind of work it does. Both issues are important when considering the overall portfolio of medical research undertaken and the Cochrane Collaboration's contribution to it.

Is it Science?

The work of the collaboration clearly involves sophisticated methods derived from science, particularly in the field of statistics. In addition, many of its contributors are researchers and scientists involved in a wide range of biomedical specialties. Science clearly requires trained scientists and the use of scientific methods; but scientific methods and particularly not exclusive statistics are frequently used in a wide range of other activities, for example, surveys and market research which would not be considered science (for a wider discussion of what constitutes science see Ref. 27). To illustrate the nature of the Collaboration's work and the contribution it makes to health, I will discuss its most celebrated systematic review in some detail, that of the anti-influenza drug Tamiflu.

The Tamiflu Saga

The Cochrane Collaboration published its first systematic review on neuraminidase inhibitors for treatment of influenza in 1999,[28] and the group updated its review in 2006.[29] The report claimed that Oseltamivir shortened symptoms of influenza and reduced complications and hospital admissions. In 2009, an outbreak of H1N1 flu in Mexico prompted governments and other health providers to purchase large stocks of neuraminidase inhibitors to have available for treatment if a major pandemic arose. In the UK, around £424 million was spent and $1.3 billion in the US.[30] The UK DH also commissioned the Cochrane collaboration to update its 2006 review at this time. Within days of starting to work on their review update the Cochrane group received a letter from Keiji Hayashi, a Japanese paediatrician challenging the reliability of the 2006 review.[31] In essence, Hayashi argued that the Cochrane group's 2006 claim that Oseltamivir reduced complications of influenza and hospital admissions was unreliable, because contrary to their assertion in the report, the group could not have extracted and analysed the data on which this claim was made since most of it was not publicly available. It transpired that the Cochrane review claim was based on a previously published meta-analysis by Kaiser *et al.*,[32] which studied 10 randomised controlled clinical trials. However, only 2 of those 10 trials were available as full peer reviewed reports, 7 of the remaining 8 were published as abstract proceedings of conferences only and one was not published at all. Furthermore neither of the 2 full publication[33,34] found evidence to support the Cochrane review claim that Tamiflu reduced complications and hospital admission. Hayashi also raised the fact that 4 of the 6 authors on the Kaiser report were employees of Hoffman–La Roche, the manufacturer of Tamiflu, and one other had been a paid consultant to the company.

The Cochrane defence in response to Hayashi's claim was that it had been misled and "duped" by its trust in the published literature.[35] However, even a brief read of the Kaiser paper makes clear that only two of the studies it included had been fully published. The statement in the 2006 Cochrane review that the authors had "extracted and analysed" all of the data on which their report was based, implied that they had access to all of these trials. The kernel of Hayashi's criticism was to expose the fact that the Cochrane group could not have done so since most of the data was not publicly available. The peer review process involved in the Kaiser paper might be criticised for publishing a weak report, but it was not misleading in describing the sources of the trials included; it was quite clear on this. On the other hand the Cochrane review does appear to have been misleading in stating that the authors had extracted and analysed all of the data included in their review; they clearly could not have done so.

In preparing for its 2009 review update, the Cochrane group requested access to all of the raw clinical trial data from Hoffman–La Roche regarding Oseltamivir. Hoffman in turn asked them to sign a confidentiality agreement. The Cochrane group declined to do this and went ahead with their 2009 review excluding all of the unpublished trials.[36] The new review withdrew the earlier claims that Oseltamivir reduced complications of influenza and hospital admissions. On the day the report was published, Hoffman–La Roche announced that it would make all of its clinical trial reports on Oseltamivir available and GlaxoSmithKline (GSK) followed suite regarding zanamivir in 2010. Subsequently, GSK sent its data to the group in early 2013 and Hoffman also did so in September that year. Activity during the intervening period is disputed; the Cochrane group mounted a very public campaign for transparency of all trial data in conjunction with the BMJ and an advocacy group, claiming that the companies were stalling, releasing incomplete data and breaking promises. The companies on the other hand claimed the delays were unavoidable, pointing out that some of the data were quite old and stored in disparate locations from which files had to be identified and retrieved. Without a confidentiality agreement, clinical data that might breach privacy had to be redacted and with over 150,000 pages to review, the whole operation involved 15–20 people working part time for three years.[35] Needless to say the Cochrane group remain sceptical. The Cochrane review update based on the newly released clinical study reports was published in April 2014.[37] This review reversed their 2006 claim that Oseltamivir reduced lower respiratory tract complications and found the data inadequate to detect an effect on pneumonia. It also updated information on side effects.

The Tamiflu saga illustrates what the Cochrane collaboration does well, the value of its contribution and its wider activity in health care. It also helps to understand what it does not do and its place in the wider context of biomedical research. Clearly, an accurate up to date review of neuraminidase inhibitors helps us to understand if and when they may be useful in managing influenza. It is also of great potential value in guiding health providers' decisions on purchasing the drug for treatment, and for stockpiling to manage future epidemics and indeed the Cochrane reviews were in fact commissioned by the UK DH for this purpose.

The Tamiflu case also illustrates that the Cochrane group is a highly effective health campaigning organisation. Its use of the medical and general media reached a wide audience and must have brought considerable pressure to bear on the companies to release their trial data. The final publication of their systematic review updates in the BMJ was accompanied by two related editorials and four viewpoint articles and two of the latter included Cochrane affiliated authors. The group undoubtedly achieved a breakthrough in improving transparency of drug company sponsored trial data and in doing so transformed what might have been a public relations disaster (their 2006 systematic review appears to have been both incompetent and misleading) into a major victory over recalcitrant big pharma. In time, I suspect the case will be best remembered for this.

It is also important to emphasise that the work undertaken by the Cochrane Collaboration is based on analysing existing data from previously published work. It does not generate any original data. None of its work seeks to test new hypotheses or to develop new knowledge. Its systematic reviews may tell us how much or little effect a treatment may have and how troublesome side effects may be compared to placebo or another drug, but it does not tell us anything new about influenza or neuraminidase inhibitors. It is best described therefore as comparative research in the sense of comparing existing sets of data and as such it is valuable for developing clinical management strategies and guiding drug purchasing. But it is not science. Comparative research, Box 3.1 studies what is already known Box 3.1, and uses standardised methods. First-hand knowledge and experience of the subject area are less important.[39] Science, Box 3.2 on the other hand explores what is previously unknown and may often have to invent new methods to do so. This distinction matters because the contributions of science and comparative research differ so much. While the latter can help us to make the best of what we already know, science seeks to understand what is currently unknown.

Box 3.1 Systematic Reviews.

1. No original hypothesis.
2. Concerned with exiting data.
3. Comparative.
4. Standard design & analysis.
5. Expertise in analytical methods required; knowledge of subject area less important.

Box 3.2 Primary Science.

1. Tests original hypothesis.
2. Seeks new knowledge.
3. Experimental.
4. Design, methods & analysis must meet experimental needs.
5. Deep knowledge of the subject area and experimental methods required.

Take for example, questions such as, is the influenza virus more or less susceptible to neuraminidase inhibitors at different stages in the natural history of infection; or is the sensitivity of the virus to such drugs related to the virulence of the strain? These are important because in retrospect the 2009 outbreak of H1N1 influenza proved to be much less virulent than feared and as a result much of the stock pile of drugs purchased was not used. But this also means that we cannot be sure how useful or not they might be should a new more virulent pandemic emerge. This was the basis for the DH's rejection of the findings of the 2014 Cochrane review when giving evidence before the House of Commons Public Accounts committee about its decision to purchase and stock pile Tamiflu. The Chief Medical Officer put forward the frequently expressed arguments regarding the limitations of systematic reviews; (i) many of the clinical trials on which the review was based were carried out during flu epidemics when many of the patients recruited may not in reality have had flu, unlike licensing studies where proof of infection was required and (ii) sub-populations of study groups may have benefited more than the overall meta-analysis indicated.[39] The urgency now is to find answers to these questions in order to clarify whether present stocks should be maintained and extended. These are important issues on which comparative research can only be silent at present in the absence of any original research data. It is the task of science to generate that information. Thus comparative research provides a snap shot of the current state of knowledge; science is concerned with adding new knowledge and understanding what we already know.

This distinction between comparative research and science is also important in relation to how they are resourced. The past three decades have seen a great expansion of comparative research in healthcare and to a large extent this has been at the expense of science and clinical science in particular, which has been in decline.[40] I have argued previously that this has been a major contributing factor to the decline in new clinical discoveries and the failure to translate new discoveries in biology into useful clinical benefits.[41] Confusion between the roles of comparative research and clinical science and conflation of the two contributed to this. As discussed in Chapter 2, Archie Cochrane was a powerful campaigner for the expansion of comparative research in collaboration with the UK DH which was seeking to extend its control of medical research (p. 120).[42] Cochrane famously derided clinical science as wasteful phenomenology, that it made no contribution to medical progress and that it should be replaced by comparative research such as systematic reviews (pp. 12, 44, 81).[2] He favoured directed research in which the investigation of novel hypotheses is replaced by managed or commissioned research following predefined protocols. This is what the collaboration named after him does and the organisation is an exemplar of the expansion of this form of comparative research. However, the growth of comparative research was facilitated by the reconfiguration of research funding in the UK resulting in a decline in support for academic medicine and clinical science,[41] which in turn contributed to undermining links between clinicians and basic science.

More recently, members of the Cochrane Collaboration have launched a new campaign to reduce waste in science, claiming that 85% of research funding is wasted because of inadequate methods of production and reporting. The campaign was launched with five consecutive articles and an editorial in the Lancet.[43-48] The authors dismissed my challenge[49] that they may not be representative of the wider biomedical community, claiming to be a mixed group including researchers in basic science and statistics.[50] There were 40 authors among the group. Their main research areas were epidemiology or public health (55%) and statistics (15%), accounting for 70% of the group. Four (10%) of the group who were engaged in clinical practice (based on publicly available CVs), all of whom had epidemiology and systematic reviews as their main research interest. Four (10%) of the group were involved in basic laboratory research. Analysis of the group's publications since 2010 identified 2,234 reports (based on PubMed searches using the authors name and location and examining article titles, abstracts and full publication as necessary to confirm ownership). Around 27% of publications were in epidemiology or public health, 23% were systematic reviews or meta analyses, 10% were clinical trials or clinical research and less than 3% were experimental basic science. The four authors identified as clinicians accounted for only 13% of the clinical science articles; most of these were accounted for by epidemiologists and statisticians among the group. Systematic reviews, opinion pieces or general reviews accounted for most (75%) of the clinicians' output and none published any basic research. Among the 4 basic scientists, 1 mainly published systematic reviews and 1 other accounted for more than half of all the experimental research articles. Interestingly, around 52% of all publications by members of the group were opinion pieces or editorials, by far its most frequent type of publication. These research interests and publications therefore are consistent with a group whose main interest is in epidemiology, public health and systematic reviews. Clinical science and basic science appear to be weakly represented and certainly not in keeping with biomedical science generally. They are also consistent with the EBM movement and the Cochrane Collaboration, not only in terms of its mission for comparative research, but also as a group heavily committed to activism, as indicated by the high output of opinion pieces and editorials.

Here I must make it clear that I do not criticise systematic reviews; they provide a valuable tool for clinicians and policy makers and this group probably do them best. However, systematic reviews differ greatly from primary science. The former is concerned with existing data. They rely on standardised methods, they do not test original hypotheses and are done by researchers with expertise in analytical tools; expertise in the subject area being less important. In contrast primary science seeks new knowledge, is experimental in nature and tests original hypotheses. Research design, methods and analytical tools must be appropriate for the experimental conditions and hypothesis being tested.

A campaign to reduce waste sounds like an obvious good, but the approach taken and knowledge and experience of the activists involved are likely to be important in determining its effectiveness. In reality determining what is wasteful in science may be more difficult than in standardised systems of research. For example, a failed experiment may seem like waste from an economic perspective, but provide valuable knowledge to a trained scientist. The difference between the two reactions will be determined by the value priorities that motivate them. To an economist focused on measuring short term utility it may appear to have no value. A scientist, on the other hand, may value the knowledge imparted by the experiment even if simply to change the direction of research. Double Nobel Prize winner Frederick Sanger described his work as a lot of luck and not getting depressed about failed experiments, as he put it, "I've had a lot of good ideas but most of them haven't worked."

An example of waste in science cited by the campaign were reports on biomarkers for cancer in 2005, of which only very few entered clinical practice.[43] But is this a justified claim? The word biomarker has been used in science to indicate the presence of biological material, specific organisms, physiological conditions or mechanisms and only first appeared in the

Oxford English Dictionary as a draft entry in 2004. It is highly likely therefore that the use of the word in reports of cancer research in 2005 may have varied in its meaning and would have appeared in articles exploring wider aspects of diseases, and their potential targets for treatment. To condemn all of this work as wasteful is absurd when considered from a scientific perspective, because it discards any knowledge gained from them without attempting to value it. This approach to waste in science essentially reflects the short term economic perspective implicit in what is currently called "needs driven research". It also identifies the EBM movement and the Cochrane Collaboration in that perspective. But this is hardly surprising since Cochrane himself used the same rhetoric to discredit clinical science as wasteful and to argue for its replacement with comparative research.

Experience, value perspectives and interests are important determinants of how waste in science is viewed and this self-selected campaign group mostly composed of researchers who have worked together collaboratively in comparative research and in other health campaigns are not representative of the wider biomedical science community. Their value perspectives regarding science may reflect this. In this context it is noteworthy that almost all of its recommendations to reduce waste involve management, monitoring and oversight, which also reflects most of the collective expertise of the group; almost nothing is mentioned about how science works best, what makes a successful science culture, how to build a science culture or how best to motivate good scientists. But this is not surprising in the absence of a strong contribution from biomedical experts with direct experience in experimental and clinical science.

Summary

The Cochrane collaboration is the most important development to arise from the EBM movement. Founded initially with support from the UK DH in 1992 it has grown to a world-wide organisation with 40,000 volunteers. The systematic reviews it produces on health interventions are valued by governments and health providers as a means to improve clinical management, design health policy and contain expenditures. That its reviews are restricted to therapeutic interventions, and its refusal to examine wider aspects of healthcare policy has been criticised and raised questions about its independence from policy makers, who are often the source of its commissioned work and funding. The collaboration knows that it faces significant challenges in relation to the efficiency of preparing reviews, its limited coverage of therapeutic areas and the debate over mission creep. It is also likely to face competition from other providers of systematic reviews.

It has shown itself to be an effective campaign group as exemplified by its efforts to achieve data transparency, which have been widely welcomed. The more recent campaign launched to reduce waste in science raises several concerns; the application of standardised methods and statistics which apply so well to comparative and commissioned research may be less applicable or counterproductive when used to critique experimental research and curiosity driven science, areas in which the group are not broadly experienced. More generally, the campaign may be seen as part of the discourse between advocates of curiosity driven science and directed research which has been running since the early 20th century. This group appears to be firmly on the side of needs driven, commissioned research reflecting its experience and interests and those of its main funders.

References

1. Cochrane AL (1931–1971). *A Critical Review with Particular Reference to the Medical Profession. In*: Medicines for the year 2000. London: Office of Health Economics, p. 2–12.
2. Cochrane A (1972). *Effectiveness and Efficiency: Random Reflections on Health Services*. London: Nuffield Provincial Trust.
3. Chalmers I (1993). The Cochrane Collaboration: Preparing, Maintaining and Disseminating Systematic Reviews of the Effects of Health Care. *Ann NY Acad Sci*, 31, 703, 156–163.
4. Starr M, Chalmers I, Clarke M (2009). The Origins, Evolution, and Future of The Cochrane Database of Systematic Reviews. *International Journal of Technology Assessment in Health Care*, 25: Supplement 1; 182–195.
5. Measuring the performance of The Cochrane Library. The Cochrane Library Oversight Committee. Available at: http://www.cochranelibrary.com/editorial/10.1002/14651858.ED000048 (Accessed on 4/12/2015).
6. Cochrane Collaboration. Annual Report & Financial Statements 2010/11. Available at: http://annual-report.cochrane.org/.
7. Oxman AD (2013). Helping People Male Well-informed Decisions about Health Care: Old and New Challenges to Achieving the Aim of the Cochrane Collaboration. *System Rev*, 2, 77.

8. The Cochrane Collaboration Annual Report & Financial Statements 2009/10. Available at: http://www.cochrane.org/sites/default/files/uploads/Annual%20 Report%202009-10_The%20Cochrane%20Collaboration.pdf.

9. Antman EM, Lau J, Kupelnick B, Mosteller F, Chalmers TC (1992). A Comparison of Results of Meta-analyses of Randomized Control Trials and Recommendations of Clinical Experts. Treatments for Myocardial Infarction. *JAMA*, 268, 240–248.

10. Smith R (2013). The Cochrane Collaboration at 20. *BMJ*, 347, 3.

11. Becker LA, Oxman AD: Chapter 22: *Overviews of Reviews*. *In* Cochrane Handbook for Systematic Reviews of Interventions Version 5.1.0 (updated March 2011). Edited by Higgins JPT, Green S. Available at: http://handbook. cochrane.org/ (Accessed on 4/12/2015).

12. Bero LA, Binder L (2013). The Cochrane Collaboration Review Prioritization Projects show that a Variety of Approaches Successfully Identify High Priority Topics. *J Clin Epidemiol*, 66, 472–473.

13. Cochrane agenda and priority setting methods group. Available at: http://priority. cochrane.org/ (Accessed 4/12/2015).

14. The James Lind Alliance. Available at: http://www.lindalliance.org/ (Accessed on 4/12/2015).

15. Tunis S (2013). Lack of Evidence for Clinical and Health Policy Decisions. *BMJ*, 347, f7155.

16. Iacobucci G (2014). The Battle for NHS111: Who Should Run it Now. *BMJ*, 348, f7659.

17. Kmietowicz Z (2014). Repeal "Intensely Damaging" Health Act, says BMA. *BMJ*, 348, g2532.

18. Moodie C, Bauld L, Stead M (2013). UK Government's Delay on Plain Tobacco Packaging: How Much Evidence is Enough? Early findings from Australia Add to a Rapidly Growing Body of Research. *BMJ*, 347, f4786.

19. Brassey J (2013). A Critique of the Cochrane Collaboration. Trip 2013. http:// blog.tripdatabase.com/2013/04/a-critique-of-cochrane-collaboration.html. (Accessed on 4/12/2015).

20. Moher D, Tsertsvadze A, Tricco AC, Eccles M, Grimshaw J, Sampson M, Barrowman N (2007). A Systematic Review Identified Few Methods and Strategies Describing when and how to Update Systematic Reviews. *J Clin Epidemiol*, 60, 1095–1104.

21. Tsafnat G, Dunn A, Glasziou P, Coiera E (2013). The Automation of Systematic Reviews. *BMJ*, 346, f139.

22. Higgins J, Churchill R, Lasserson T, Chandler J, Tovey D (2012). Update from the Methodological Expectations of Cochrane Intervention Reviews (MECIR) project. *In*: Cochrane methods, (Eds.). Chandler J, Clarke M, Higgins J.

Chichester, UK: John Wiley & Sons. Available at: http://www.thecochranelibrary. com/SpringboardWebApp/userfiles/ccoch/file/Files/coch_Method_2012% 5B1%5D.pdf (Accessed on 4/12/2015).

23. Glasziou PP1, Shepperd S, Brassey J (2010). Can We Rely on the Best Trial? A Comparison of Individual Trials and Systematic Reviews. *BMC Med Res Methodol*, 10, 23.

24. Hemens BJ, Haynes RB McMaster (2012). Premium LiteratUre Service (PLUS) Performed Well for Identifying New Studies for Updated Cochrane Reviews. *J Clin Epidemiol*, 65(1), 62–72.

25. Sagliocca L1, De Masi S, Ferrigno L, Mele A, Traversa G (2013). A Pragmatic Strategy for the Review of Clinical Evidence. *J Eval Clin Pract*, 19(4), 689–696.

26. Guyatt GH (1991). Evidence-based medicine (Editorial). American College of Physicians Journal Club. *Ann Intern Med*, 114 (Suppl. 2), A16.

27. Sheridan DJ (2012). The Rise and Fall of Medical Science in the 20th Century. *In*: Medical Science in the 21st Century; Sunset or New Dawn. London: Imperial College Press.

28. Jefferson T, Demicheli V, Deeks J, Rivetti D (1999). Neuraminidase Inhibitors for Preventing and Treating Influenza in Healthy Adults. *Cochrane Database Syst Rev*, 2, CD001265.

29. Jefferson T, Demicheli V, Rivetti D, Jones M, Di Pietrantonj C, Rivetti A (2006). Antivirals for influenza in healthy adults: systematic review. *Lancet*, 367, 303–313.

30. Jack A (2014). Tamiflu: A Nice Little Earner. *BMJ*, 348, g2524.

31. Hayashi K. Hayashi's criticism on previous Cochrane review. Available at: http://www.bmj.com/content/suppl/2009/12/07/bmj.b5106.DC1/jeft726562. ww1_default.pdf (Accessed on 4/12/2015).

32. Kaiser L1, Wat C, Mills T, Mahoney P, Ward P, Hayden F (2003). Impact of Oseltamivir Treatment on Influenza-related Lower Respiratory Tract Complications and Hospitalizations. *Arch Intern Med*, 163(14), 1667–1672.

33. Treanor JJ, Hayden FG, Vrooman PS, Barbarash R, Bettis R, Riff D, Singh S, Kinnersley N, Ward P, Mills RG (2000). Efficacy and Safety of the Oral Neuraminidase Inhibitor Oseltamivir in Treating Acute Influenza: A Randomized Controlled Trial. US Oral Neuraminidase Study Group. *JAMA*, 283(8), 1016–1024.

34. Nicholson KG1, Aoki FY, Osterhaus AD, Trottier S, Carewicz O, Mercier CH, Rode A, Kinnersley N, Ward P (2000). Efficacy and Safety of Oseltamivir in Treatment of Acute Influenza: A Randomised Controlled Trial. Neuraminidase Inhibitor Flu Treatment Investigator Group. *Lancet*, 355(9218), 1845–1850.

35. Belluz J (2014). Tug of War for Antiviral Drugs Data Julia Belluz hears from both sides in the Lengthy Battle between the Drug Giants and Researchers that led to the Release of Full Clinical Trial Data on Neuraminidase Inhibitors. Does the Release of these Files Herald a more Transparent Era? *BMJ*, 348, g2227.

36. Jefferson T, Jones M, Doshi P, Del Mar C (2009). Neuraminidase Inhibitors for Preventing and Treating Influenza in Healthy Adults: Systematic Review and Metaanalysis. *BMJ*, 339, b5106.

37. Jefferson T, Jones M, Doshi P, Spencer EA, Onakpoya I, Heneghan CJ (2014). Oseltamivir for Influenza in Adults and Children: Systematic Review of Clinical Study Reports and Summary of Regulatory Comments. *BMJ*, 348, g2545.

38. Gøtzsche PC, Ioannidis JP (2012). Content Area Experts as Authors: Helpful or Harmful for Systematic Reviews and Meta-analyses? *BMJ*, 345, e7031.

39. CMO Defends Decision to Stockpile Tamiflu and Says She Would Do it Again. *BMJ*, 2014, 349, 4.

40. Sheridan, D (2006). Reversing the Decline of Academic Medicine in Europe. *The Lancet*, 367, 1698–1701.

41. Sheridan DJ (2012). *The Decline of Biomedical Science Despite Unprecedented Technological Advances: A 21st century paradox. In* Medical Science in the 21st century; sunset or new dawn. London: Imperial College Press.

42. Sheard S, Donaldson L (2006). The nations Doctor; the role of the chief medical officer. Oxford: Radcliffe publishing, 1855–1998.

43. Macleod MR, Michie S, Roberts I, Dirnagl U, Chalmers I, Ioannidis JPA, Salman RA, Chan AW, Glasziou P (2014). Biomedical Research: Increasing Value, Reducing Waste. *Lancet*, 383, 101–104.

44. Ioannidis JPA, Greenland S, Hlatky MA, Khoury MJ, Macleod MR, Moher D, Schulz KF, Tibshiranim R (2014). Research: Increasing Value, Reducing Waste 2 Increasing Value and Reducing Waste in Research Design, Conduct, and Analysis. *Lancet*, 383, 166–175.

45. Al-Shahi Salman R, Beller E, Kagan J, Hemminki E, Phillips RS, Savulescu J, Macleod M, Wisely J, Chalmers I (2014). Research: Increasing Value, Reducing Waste 3 Increasing Value and Reducing Waste in Biomedical Research Regulation and Management. *Lancet*, 383, 176–185.

46. Chalmers I, Bracken MB, Djulbegovic B, Garattini S, Grant J, Gülmezoglu AM, Howells DW, Ioannidis JPA, Oliver S (2014). Research: Increasing Value, Reducing Waste 1 How to Increase Value and Reduce Waste when Research Priorities are Set. *Lancet*, 383, 156–165.

47. Glasziou P, Altman DG, Bossuyt P, Boutron I, Clarke M, Julious S, Michie S, Moher D, Wager E (2014). Research: Increasing Value, Reducing Waste 5

Reducing Waste from Incomplete or Unusable Reports of Biomedical Research. *Lancet*, 383, 267–276.

48. An-Wen Chan, Fujian (2014). Research: Increasing Value, Reducing Waste 4 Increasing Value and Reducing Waste: Addressing Inaccessible Research. *Lancet*, 383, 257–266.

49. Sheridan DJ (2014). Research: Increasing Value, Reducing Waste. *Lancet*, 383, 1123.

50. Paul Glasziou, Malcolm R Macleod, Iain Chalmers, John PA Ioannidis, Rustam Al-Shahi Salman, An-Wen Chan (2014). Research: Increasing Value, Reducing Waste. *Lancet*, 383, 1126.

Chapter 4

Evidence-Based Medicine and the Evolution of Health Related Research

Historical Context

The evidence-based medicine (EBM) movement was launched as a campaign by a group mainly composed of clinical epidemiologists seeking to promote medical practice and teaching that is more aligned with the best and most up to date research evidence. It appeared ostensibly as a spontaneous initiative arising from a group of clinicians and academics; however, this would be an oversimplification of its origins. The movement has been exceptionally successful in establishing its presence in health care and now occupies a unique position as a provider of information aimed at assisting clinical practice as well as furthering the needs of health care providers. It also fulfils a long cherished aspiration of health service mandarins to develop health services research [also referred to as health related research] to assist the implementation of health policies. As discussed in Chapters 2 and 3, the EBM movement has wide international support. However, it is strongest in the UK where it was recognised by and provided with initial funding by the Department of Health (DH) as a form of health related research closely aligned with government health policy. In order to understand how it has come to occupy such an important place in health systems today and the reasons behind its meteoric rise, it needs to be considered in the historical context of how health care and medical science have evolved over the past century. Much of what has been written about the history of this period tends to focus on the politics and personal relations of those involved.[8] Almost all of this has been written from a perspective of social science and public health interests closely aligned to the DH. These included some commissioned by the DH,[1] at its invitation,[2] from Social Science Units supported by it over several decades[3] or under the auspices of the Nuffield Trust. This chapter will therefore focus on the evolution of science and health policy in the UK, how this consolidated the evidence-based medicine movement and how it impacted on medicine and medical science more widely.

The Haldane Principle

The Haldane Principle is named after Viscount Haldane who chaired the Machinery of Government Committee, which was set up in 1917 as a sub-committee of the Reconstruction Committee to enquire into and recommend changes to improve the functions of various government departments.[4] When discussing research, the Haldane committee noted that the Medical Research Committee, a forerunner of the Medical Research Council (MRC), had been constituted in 1911 on the basis of funds provided by parliament, equivalent to one penny in respect of every insured person, amounting to £50,000–£60,000 annually. It was recognised that these funds were not to be restricted for the study of any particular disease or for the purpose of investigating questions suggested by the administrators of the National Insurance Act, but rather for the study of all aspects of medical practice and theory. The committee was at some pains to set out that the research conducted by the MRC was not for the immediate purposes of any particular administrative department and that the minister to whom it was accountable did not set or suggest the areas to be investigated (p. 28).[4] Instead, a separate Advisory Council consisting of "men of science" was appointed for that purpose. In this matter, the committee was quite particular in its use of language to make clear its intention that the work supported by the MRC should be free of political interference.

The Haldane committee did not attempt to enunciate the concept of science free from political interference as an explicit "principle" and its report did not use that word; that label was later used by Lord Hailsham when referring to the Haldane report in a party political debate in the House of Commons in 1964. This has led to an historical dispute over the appropriateness of the word "principle" in relation to Haldane's report.[5] The argument is that because this word does not appear in the Haldane report, the concept of a Haldane principle was merely a historical invention. This is then used without reference to what the Haldane report actually contained in order to refute its recommendation that science should be free from administrative interference. Lord Rothschild would later use this as the basis of his dismissal of the concept of scientific freedom in 1972.

Haldane was a successful barrister and politician and he was interested in education, having been involved in founding both Imperial College, and The London School of Hygiene and Tropical Medicine. He was also familiar with philosophical thought and translated works by Hagel and Schopenhauer. It seems likely therefore that he would have understood how knowledge is acquired and the distinction between enquiries relating to established areas of knowledge and those seeking to discover new knowledge. This is important because later commentators would seek to discount this distinction in order to justify conflating all forms of enquiry as being of a similar character so as to support their being supervised by a single administrative authority.

In outlining its views on research and information, Haldane's committee referred to enquiries under three categories: those carried out (a) within administrative departments, (b) under the supervision of administrative departments and (c) research carried out for the general use of administrative departments, but under the supervision of separate authorities not charged with administrative responsibilities. The language used suggests that Haldane's committee intended to distinguish between different forms of enquiry and that it recognised science as a unique exploratory endeavour at the frontier of knowledge unlike other forms of enquiry in areas of established knowledge. When commenting on the MRC, the Haldane report placed the work of the MRC firmly in category (c) and drew an "important distinction" between the research carried out by the MRC "and all other work carried out within the sphere of the department". In its first annual report, members of the MRC did in fact acknowledge the "remarkable freedom" they were afforded in bringing "flexible and rapid assistance to the national need on occasions of emergency with the least possible delay".

Medical Research Council

The independence of the Medical Research Committee and later Council (MRC) was maintained under the direction of Walter Morley Fletcher who was appointed as its secretary in 1914 and remained so until 1933. Fletcher had been a successful physiological scientist at Cambridge and was elected to the Royal Society in 1915. He strenuously defended the independence of the MRC, and in this he was strongly supported by the permanent Secretary of the DH, Robert Morant and by Christopher Addison. Addison was a Doctor and Professor of Anatomy at Sheffield before moving to London, where he taught at Charing Cross Hospital. He later entered politics and became Minister of Munitions in 1916, of Reconstruction in 1917, and Minister for Health in 1919. Addison strongly supported the Haldane committee's recommendations that the direction of scientific research should be left to scientists and be independent of administrative interference in a memorandum on the organisation of medical research.[6] Like Haldane he recognised that the DH would also need to carry out research to meet its policy objectives, but that the inevitable bias implicit in this would risk undermining the rigour of scientific work. For this reason, he urged that the latter should be research driven under the supervision of scientists.

Having secured the necessary resources and political backing, the MRC prospered and succeeded in setting up a world class biomedical science infrastructure in the UK under Fletcher's leadership. It is clear that Fletcher's ambitions extended widely to establish biomedical science in the UK, and the MRC was the principal means to achieve this. In this he had a major impact on the development of bacteriology, virology and immunology as well as on physiology, pathology and biochemistry. Through his position, he was able to influence several major philanthropic donations in favour of this objective; for example he was instrumental in convincing the Dunn Trustees to establish the Dunn Institute of Biochemistry at Cambridge and the Dunn School of Pathology at Oxford. He also persuaded the Rockefeller Foundation to establish an institute of Biochemistry at Oxford and a School of Pathology at Cambridge.[8] His success reflected his skilled administrative abilities and he clearly operated in a rather narrow context of his friendships and academic loyalties, especially in relation to Cambridge.[7] In today's world this might be seen as patronage and a tinge of cronyism, but was probably unremarkable in his time.

The work of the MRC was of course evolving in the area of health, in which other interests were active. There were difficulties between the MRC and all of these interests at one time or another. For example, the Cancer Committee set up by the ministry in 1923 led to tension which was resolved in an agreement between Fletcher and Sir George Newman, the Chief Medical Officer the following year. This set out that the ministry would focus on research in the interests of public health, applied knowledge and medical services.[8] Fletcher also came into conflict with the medical profession and the Royal Colleges in particular. He was as keen to protect the direction of scientific enquiry from interference from the leaders of the profession as he was from ministerial departments and argued that clinicians had a poor record in supervising research. When the British Empire Cancer Campaign was launched in 1923, like many others,[9] he saw it as competing with the already established Imperial Cancer Research Fund and argued that solving the problem of cancer required highly trained biological scientists and was beyond what could be achieved in a clinical arena. He was alarmed by the Leverhulme Trust's donation to the Royal College of Physicians which allowed it to establish research scholarships; he vigorously opposed clinicians getting involved in "controlling research" because he felt they were not trained as scientists and had little experience in supervising research. This involved him in bitter tensions with Lords Dawson and Moynihan,[8] Presidents of the Royal College of Physicians and Surgeons. Despite this, Fletcher and the MRC were committed to and strongly motivated by the belief[10] that basic medical science would lead to improvements in national health. The main difficulty as he saw it was that most clinicians had little or no training in scientific methods which Fletcher believed was essential to supervise research. In fact, great efforts were made by the MRC in the following years to correct this deficiency.

Medical Research

At the beginning of the 20th century, clinical science was virtually nonexistent in UK medical schools and had much catching up to do. For an excellent review of this period, see Ref. 11. There were no full time clinical professors and little clinical experimental work in the universities. Germany had a strong tradition in academic medicine and this had influenced the leaders of the new John Hopkins Medical School in the US to follow the same path when it was founded in 1889. Sir William Osler had come from John Hopkins to take up the post of Regius Professor of Medicine at Oxford in 1907 and was highly critical of the conditions he found. In giving evidence to the Royal Commission on University Education in London in 1913, he and others condemned the absence of a clinical laboratory base in the London Medical Schools and the lack of links with the universities. This led to the commission's recommendation to develop academic professorial units in the London Teaching Hospitals (p. 121).[12] By 1914, the MRC already had plans to develop its first clinical academic unit having identified suitable candidates in TR Elliot and Thomas Lewis and found a solution to the problem of access to hospital beds.[13] With the outbreak of the WWI these plans had to be postponed and priority given to medical problems related to the war. However, the MRC did go ahead in appointing Lewis to investigate and develop methods for managing the problem of "soldier's heart" and distinguishing it from other known cardiac pathology.[14] Through this and its support for other war related problems such as investigating the effects of toxic gases, the MRC had gained an important voice in planning clinical research by the end of the war. This experience is also likely to have influenced the MRC's decision to support the establishment of clinical research and experimental medicine in close relation to universities. Thomas Lewis' appointment in 1916 at University College Hospital with close links to the Cardiographic Department in the medical school and access to beds was the first example of this. By 1925, professorial chairs of medicine had been established in five London medical schools and during the 1920s, the MRC had provided grants to all of these as well as to the units at St Andrews, Edinburgh and Sheffield.[11]

In 1930, Sir Thomas Lewis identified that a lack of trained clinical researchers hampered the development of clinical science[15] and called for an institute to achieve this. The MRC did not agree to provide an institute but did accept the need to provide studentships and fellowships in clinical research. During the 1930s, there was much tension about the direction of clinical research and how it should be supervised; the presidents of the Royal Colleges complained passionately about a lack of support for it and the failure to incorporate new knowledge gained in biology to advance surgical and medical practice.[16] This reflected differences in how clinical research should be supervised. Fletcher and the MRC believed that clinical research departments should be based in the universities with links to clinical services and was critical of the ability of clinicians to supervise research without such support.[10] In reality, both sides were agreed on the principle that progress needed close links between clinicians and basic scientists as Lord Moynihan made clear in his comments;[16] his complaint was that progress in physiology was not leading to advances in medicine because the two were not well integrated. It is ironic that this problem would re-emerge in the 21st century as "the translation gap"[17] due to medicine once again becoming increasingly separate from biomedical science. Back in the 1930s, the challenge was met by founding clinical research units, initially in London, Oxford, Cambridge and Edinburgh. Progress was interrupted by WWII but continued after it.

The National Health Service (NHS)

The NHS Act in 1946 profoundly changed health care and clinical research in the UK. DH became responsible for all hospital beds and also took on an important role in clinical research. In order to establish a mechanism for the latter, a joint committee of the MRC and the DH was convened in 1951 under the chairmanship of Sir Henry Cohen. The main recommendations of its report, published in 1953 and accepted by the MRC and DH in 1957 were that (a) the MRC would supervise and manage the organisation of clinical research in close collaboration with the DH, (b) that research units would be decentralised to regional hospital boards, (c) research would be closely linked to medical practice and free of administrative interference and (d) clinical research staff would hold honorary appointments equivalent to full time practicing staff.[18,19] This led to expansion of clinical research units across the country and was assisted by the establishment of the Clinical Research Board by the MRC in 1953 until it was disbanded in 1974. The change was particularly noted by Sir Raymond Hoffenberg, who had spent some time in London in the 1950s, later immigrating to the UK in 1968 supported by the MRC. He was well placed to observe how clinical research was no longer limited to research centres but was evident in all clinical institutions.[20] Arguably the most important reason for this was the support for clinical research by the NHS in implementing recommendations of the Cohen report. This made academic medicine more attractive to young clinicians and provided clinical services including hospital beds to support clinical research. A crucial aspect of this was the "knock for knock" arrangement between the DH and Education and Science whereby some costs related to clinical research and academic salaries were reimbursed between the NHS and Universities in recognition of clinical service work and teaching by clinical academics. This was perhaps a golden age for clinical research in the UK, as one witness described it "The Health Departments at that stage were all for clinical research".[21] During the 1960s and 1970s, clinical research flourished and advances in all specialties were made. Many advances required new and specialised skills which led to the development of the medical specialties of neurology, cardiology, gastroenterology, endocrinology, respiratory medicine, psychiatry, etc. Academic specialists departments also began to appear at this time.

Medical Progress, Increasing Complexity and Costs

This was also a period in which diagnosis and treatment of many diseases improved rapidly. Understanding of the causes of acute coronary heart disease advanced rapidly from the late 1950s and heralded the introduction of a wide range of diagnostic methods and treatments. Coupled with better understanding of methods for prevention, this led to a dramatic reduction in heart attacks and deaths over the following decades.[22] Similar progress was made in almost all areas of medicine and surgery. Collaboration with scientists in other fields led to the introduction of new imaging techniques based on ultrasound and magnetic resonance, while progress in computers and electronics led to the development of CT scans. Each of these depended on new discoveries in fields a long way from the bed side, but understanding of their diagnostic use and their application in medicine was made possible by close collaboration between natural scientists and clinicians, radiologists and pathologists. Development of new treatments also accelerated from the rediscovery of aspirin as an important anti-thrombotic agent for preventing heart attacks to the discovery of β-blockers and a range of safer and more effective anti-hypertensive drugs, histamine-2 antagonists for treating peptic ulcers and many others. The introduction of antibiotics transformed the way infections were treated and dramatically improved prognosis for common infections such as pneumonia. Cancer treatments also improved; although few cures would become available survival rates did improve significantly. Indeed, the period from 1955 to 1980 was probably one in which clinical medicine advanced more rapidly than any other in recent history.

Many of these advances increased the complexity of medicine and accelerated specialisation, particularly in hospital medicine. They also led to increasing health care costs and this in turn caused concerns about future sustainability among health funders. The question of cost-effectiveness of new methods of treatment became increasingly important. The case of coronary care units was a celebrated example of this. Coronary care units, by providing clinical scientist's access to patients with acute coronary heart disease, made a great contribution to better understanding of the natural history of the disease and in turn in paving the way for further progress in diagnosis and treatment as discussed in Chapter 2. Attempts to compare crude mortality outcomes for hospital versus home treatment became highly controversial for two reasons; clinicians were concerned that randomisation would be difficult, which proved to be correct and because simple mortality comparisons ignored the scientific benefits contributed by such units in understanding the disease. Almost inevitably tensions developed between the aspirations of practicing clinicians including those academics who were interested in investigating the conditions they were treating and the needs for research as viewed by those responsible for managing the health service. The former saw the need to find better diagnostic methods and treatments for the diseases afflicting their patients, whereas those charged with running the service had long sought to establish research to measure the performance and cost effectiveness of the service as a whole and to improve its effectiveness. / The Nuffield Trust published a series of essays setting out the perspectives on health needs as viewed by the DH during the 1960s and 1970s, see for example, Refs. 23–25. These are focused almost exclusively on issues related to health economics, public health, social medicine, but strikingly devoid of contributions related to clinical or academic medicine. The emphasis was on rising costs, often with veiled criticism of medical advances (pp. xviii–xix),[24] as failing to solve problems for which they were in fact never intended. Discussion of medical conditions when included was often limited to over-simplified reviews with little expert input (pp. 71–77).[25] By this time, it was clear that the enthusiasm for clinical research which had been a feature of the NHS from the late 1950s had waned. Clinical research had been a factor in driving up health costs and the need to better understand how this occurred and to find ways to optimise cost effectiveness were becoming urgent issues. This led to a change in research priorities as viewed by the DH, and to the concept of needs driven research, which it was argued would be better met in other directions, principally in public health, health economics and social medicine.

Health Services Research

Up until 1960, the NHS had little capacity to undertake research independently. It became clear that this lack was limiting its ability to manage rising costs and the hospital building programme. Sir George Godber, appointed Chief Medical Officer in 1960, understood this and initiated efforts to develop a research programme. He persuaded Dr Richard Cohen, who had been Secretary to the MRC, to move to the DH as his deputy to fulfill this objective. By the early 1970s, 10 units had been set up to undertake health service research, mainly in the field of public health, which included social medicine, pathology, addiction, psychiatry, community medicine, epidemiology and organisational research for which an additional 43 project grants had been awarded.[25] Some of these units continued to undertake research principally in order to meet academic peer review standards, while others were more concerned with research relevant to the DH. Some maintained close links to the DH while maintaining joint appointments with the hospital in which they were situated; of these, the unit at St Thomas Hospital headed by Prof Walter Holland was foremost.[3] It seems clear that the Department's interest in research did not include support for traditional clinical research; rather there was concern "not to leave research into the value and management of new advances to the chance interest of others with no service responsibilities".[26] Indeed, it seems to have been the case that clinical research had come to be viewed as a problem for the Department. As discussed in Chapter 2, Dr Cohen was closely linked to Archie Cochrane and instigated his invitation from the Nuffield Trust to give the Carling Lecture in 1972, in which he mounted his attack on clinical medicine and clinical science. The development of coronary care units to manage patients with heart attacks involved a significant increase in ward running costs and was of concern to the Department;[27] Cochrane's extraordinary rhetoric on this subject and on cardiologists in general was a clear signal of challenging times ahead for clinical medicine.[28] Cochrane's "battle for coronary care units" based on his premature analysis that they were not cost effective discouraged the introduction of CCUs in the UK but failed to stop their development more widely and the immense contribution they made to the decline in cardiac morbidity and mortality over the following decades. Of course, cardiac medicine did become substantially more expensive to deliver as treatments available advanced. This failure to control the spread of expensive new treatments may have contributed to the view that research leading to advances in care which were contributing to rising costs was a threat to health care and that it needed to be controlled.[29] The obvious way to achieve this would be to change the way research was planned by taking it out of the hands of those who delivered care and therefore would be more likely to prioritise deficiencies in diagnosis and treatment and put it under the control of those charged with managing the service as a whole.

Medical Research and Health Policy

The drive for more central control of research to meet policy needs had been growing throughout government during the 1960s and led to an inquiry chaired by Sir Burke Trend which reported in 1963.[30] Trend held the position of cabinet secretary, one of the most important positions in UK government, and was very highly regarded at home and abroad; Henry Kissinger said of him "he made the cabinet ministers he served appear more competent than they could possibly be". The Trend report maintained that the concept set out by Haldane in 1918[4] should be continued, whereby research should be free from interference from administrative departments. Despite this, independence of the research councils would not endure for much longer. Trend did little to allay ministerial concerns that more research was needed to support policy initiatives and a further report was commissioned by the Secretary of State for Education and Science, chaired by Lord Heyworth, which reported in 1965.[31] This centred on the role that Social Science could and should play in supporting government policy and the relative lack of such research in the UK. It recommended strengthening research in this area to support government policy and recommended that this should be done through a new Social Science Research Council (SSRC) in order to maintain autonomy from ministerial influence. This was accepted by the government in 1965 and the SSRC received its Royal Charter. Although the Heyworth committee maintained the research independent approach recommended by Trend, and Haldane, this would change radically in just a few years with the Rothschild inquiry.

The Rothschild Report

In 1970, Edward Heath became Prime Minister and the government published a white paper on the reorganisation of central government with the objective of ensuring clearly defined accountability and responsibility across departments in order improve formulation of policy. One outcome was the commissioning of Lord Rothschild to chair an inquiry into government research and development. Rothschild was the head of The Central Policy Review Staff, an independent unit within the cabinet office set up by Heath, to assist coordination of policy across government departments. He had formerly been Head of research at Royal Dutch Shell and Chairman of the Agricultural Research Council, having trained as a Physiologist and been elected a Fellow of the Royal Society. In his 1971 report,[32] Lord Rothschild proposed the most radical shake-up of science administration the UK had seen in 50 years. His report took a management perspective of research and development (R&D), the position as it might be viewed by a director of R&D. His focus was on the need to make the government's R&D programme more efficient with better management systems and accountability. For this reason issues such as how much research was being done and should be done, what was the right balance between fundamental and applied research, what were the important research priorities and what systems were in place to evaluate the R&D programme were all dismissed as irrelevant or unanswerable. He argued that the funder of research ultimately had to resolve these questions based on what was affordable, if necessary with the advice from scientists and other experts. He argued further that, the key issue to be decided was the overall portfolio of research required by government and that scientists, engineers and other experts were not in a position to hold reliable views on this. This led him to conclude that all applied research should be done on a "customer–contractor basis". The customer orders the research and the contractor provides it. He acknowledged the argument that fundamental research can, through chance observations, be just as important but argued that the country's needs could not be left to such a form of "scientific roulette". He then argued that, since much of the research done by the Medical, Agricultural and Natural Environment Research councils was applied, it should be commissioned and approved by the relevant departments as its customers.

Rothschild's report dismissed the concepts of scientific independence as laid down by Haldane and Addison and reaffirmed by Trend and Heyworth. In doing so, Rothschild was quite clear in his view that scientific independence had "little or no bearing on the conduct and management of Government R&D in the '70s". He did, however, acknowledge that an amount of general research was usually needed in undertaking applied research and estimated that this would amount to around 10% of the contract budget and be disbursed at the discretion of the controller of R&D. Rothschild acknowledged that his proposals would place a new management burden on government departments and recommended that a new post of Chief Scientific Advisor should be established with appropriate support to undertake this work. This meant that funds previously allocated to the research councils should now be transferred to the relevant government departments which would then disburse the funds back to the councils in respect of specific contracts. These would attract a surcharge to cover the expense of basic or curiosity driven research required to fulfill the contracts stated objectives.

The White Paper which led to the Rothschild report also stimulated a second inquiry. This was appointed by the Council for Scientific Policy and approved by the Secretary of State for Education and Science, Margaret Thatcher. It was chaired by Sir Frederick Dainton, who sat with four high ranking scientists with a strong background in discovery in physics, chemistry and geology and was charged with reviewing the future of the research council system.[33] The Dainton report recognised that government departments must be closely involved in formulating research policy and that some organisational changes were needed to improve this. It also recommended that the individual research councils worked well and could not be effectively replaced by a single monolithic national research council. It insisted that the independence of the councils should be preserved in relation to scientific responsibilities and scientific merit. In order to improve coordination with government policy, Dainton proposed the establishment of a Board of Research Councils which would comprise the heads of the Research Councils, the President of the Royal Society, a Vice-Chancellor, and representatives from the Cabinet office and other ministries.

The recommendations of both reports were largely accepted by government in 1972. Rothschild's principle of the customer–contractor was adopted and Dainton's recommendation to maintain the research councils was also accepted as was his proposal for a supervisory board.[34] Reaction from the science community to the Rothschild proposals was almost entirely hostile,[35–38] but with some exceptions.[39] The objections were all along predictable lines. Curiosity driven research could not be easily commissioned by contractors and without it "man will retrogress". Rothschild's calculations were claimed to be inaccurate and the time scale for consultation was held to be so short that the outcome was a foregone conclusion. Government departments, it was argued, lacked the experience and ability to direct R&D. Research council representatives were almost exclusively opposed to Rothschild. Support for Rothschild came mainly from social scientists and economists, primarily based on the argument that basic science is not cost effective and does not adequately meet the overall needs of society. Professor Harvey Brooks, Dean of the School of Engineering at Harvard praised aspects of the customer–contractor principle which had been used in the US since the mid-1940s, but then went on to outline a long list of its deficiencies.[39] An immediate and important consequence of the acceptance of the customer–contractor principle was that ministries found themselves responsible for a substantial body of applied R&D. To facilitate this they were to receive a percentage of funds previously allocated to the research councils. Rothschild had recommended that this should be about 50%, but in the event after much discussion and debate, 18% increasing to 35% over 3 years out of a total budget of £56.4 million would be transferred from the 3 councils involved. In the case of the MRC this amounted to a loss of £2.25 million in the first year rising to £5.5 million out of a total budget of £22.4 million in 1971–1972.[40] In addition, each department was to appoint a Chief Scientific Adviser.

Sir John Gray, Secretary to the MRC from 1968 to 1977, recounted the background to the commissioning of the Rothschild report.[41] One morning in October 1970, he and the other Research Council secretaries with the Chairman of the Council of Scientific Policy were called urgently to a meeting at the Department of Education and Science. The purpose was to review the future of the Councils which was due to be discussed in cabinet that day and the minister, Margaret Thatcher wanted to be briefed on it. At the time the research councils were believed to be at risk of being disbanded, particularly the Agricultural Research Council following an internal civil service report by Sir Paul Osmond. The councils' leaders had decided to stand together as a group to resist being dismantled. Gray reports that Margaret Thatcher agreed and successfully resisted implementation of the Osmond report; however, there was an important caveat. Sir Frederick Dainton, Chairman of the Council of Scientific Policy was asked to consult and prepare a report and in addition a final report from an independent person was to be commissioned. That person would be Lord Rothschild.

Rothschild in Reverse

Although Rothschild had recommended the transfer of funds from the MRC to the DH, the MRC continued to resist in terms of the amount to be transferred in the months following the report's publication. One example of this was the case of molecular biology, which one side argued was fundamental research while the other believed it all related to disease and was therefore applied. The MRC successfully claimed it was "strategic" rather than applied and therefore should remain within its remit. The DH appointed Dr Richard Cohen as its first Chief Scientific Advisor in 1972. Cohen had been deputy Chief Medical Officer and was previously a medical officer at the MRC. However, he had little experience as a scientist and indeed the Department was not well equipped to take on the role it was given by Rothschild. Sir Patrick Nairne who became permanent secretary to the DHSS in 1975 recalled that when he took up his post a review of MRC activity was still on going with the objective of linking NHS priorities to particular parts of the MRC programme so that the funds it had been allocated could be directed to them. In reality, little direct commissioning by the DHSS took place.[42] Douglas Black who followed Cohen as Chief Scientific Advisor in 1973 initiated a study to determine priorities in medical research based on the burden of disease,[43] which greatly assisted the process of allocating funds by the

DHSS in support of MRC work.[42] This system continued to operate during the 1970s aided by closer relations between the MRC and members of the DHSS. In reality, therefore the system which evolved had much less impact on the MRC than it had feared. Most of its support for research continued as before but with the added exercise of fitting it into DHSS priority categories. It was also clear that the MRC remained adamant that the funds transferred to the DHSS should be returned to it and Douglas Black was not unsympathetic to this.[43] By the late 1970s, it seems that the DHSS itself came to see these arrangements as bureaucratic, burdensome and unproductive.[44] At this time, the Public Accounts Committee decided to investigate the outcome of the transfer of funds between the MRC and the DHSS. Evidence was taken from both sides with the MRC making a strong case that the funds should be returned to it,[42] while the DHSS case may have been weakened by some loss of confidence in the process which had evolved.[44] In the event, it seems that the committee also took the view that the commissioning process was artificial, bureaucratic and burdensome and served little purpose. The committee's report concluded that there was little point in continuing the commissioning arrangements[45] and the new government agreed in 1981 to return most of the transferred funds.[46,47]

The DHSS reaction to the reversal of Rothschild's recommendation was ambiguous. The Chief Medical Officer, Henry Yellowlees felt that the transferred funds had given the DHSS an important degree of influence over health research. However, the Chief Scientific Advisor, Sir Arthur Buller was less convinced that such influence could be usefully employed (p. 58)[44] and Sir Patrick Nairne who was the Accounting Officer as well as Permanent Secretary spoke in support of the MRC's view, having come to believe the prioritising procedures developed in the DHSS served little useful purpose and were burdensome (p. 82).[2] An account of the DHSS work to implement the Rothschild proposals shows that great efforts were made, including the appointment of a chief scientific advisor and an accounting officer as well as establishing a complex committee structure (p. 18).[2] These efforts, however, appear to have been strong on bureaucratic and management processes, but relatively weak in understanding the biomedical science it was supposed to procure. There were several reasons for this. Social Science, health economic and public health interests tended to dominate the DHSS, particularly the Chief Scientists Research Committee (pp. 61–63)[2] and were less familiar with and sympathetic to original exploratory science. There was undoubtedly a competitive atmosphere between those committed to natural sciences, and social sciences and differences in the use of language, rhetoric and logic in natural science and social sciences may have exacerbated the difficulties. On the one hand, the natural sciences were often accused of scientific snobbery (p. 65)[3] while many in natural sciences questioned whether social science may have been too closely aligned to civil power and of being too biddable.[48] The concordat arrived at between the DHSS and the MRC returned the funds which had been transferred following the Rothschild report to the latter. This had a number of predictable added effects; it reduced tension between them, which allowed more effective collaboration, giving the DHSS better representation in the MRC. However, the reverse did not occur to the same degree, and as a result the long standing aspirations within the DHSS to develop an internal programme of health services research was less hindered by competing influences from natural sciences and academic medicine. A further effect was that despite reversal of the Rothschild funds transfer, his customer–contractor principle was maintained within the DHSS and implemented with less distraction. As a result, units which had previously been supported by the DHSS on a fairly informal basis came under a more rigorous regime.[2]

NHS Reforms

The 1980s also heralded the beginning of a period of reform resulting in unprecedented changes in the NHS. The range and extensive nature of these reforms on looking back now seems staggering; each represented a nationwide restructuring of different aspects of the health service, see Box 4.1. They undoubtedly reflect deep concerns among policy makers about the sustainability of the service, some even amounting to reversal of previous reforms introduced just a few years earlier as in the abolition of Family Health Service Authorities in 1994, just four years after they were established. Not surprisingly they also proved immensely disruptive for medical research. This was especially so in the case of the introduction of general management as recommended by the Griffiths Report. Sir Roy Griffiths was a businessman commissioned by Margaret Thatcher to report on the management of the health service in 1983. His recommendation that general managers should be introduced throughout the NHS was accepted and had a major effect on the way

Box 4.1   National Health Service Reforms Since 1980.

1. 1980 Health Services Act: Care in the Community.
2. 1982 Abolition of Area Health Authorities.
3. 1983 Griffith's Report: Introduction of General Managers throughout NHS.
4. 1885 Hospital Complaints Procedure Act.
5. 1985 Project 2000: Transforms Nursing Education.
6. 1985 NHS Management Board Established.
7. 1987 Hospital Episodes Statistics introduced; data available from 1989.
8. 1987 Hospital Staffing: Achieving a Balance.
9. 1988 DH and Department of Social Security split.
10. 1988 House of Lords Select committee on Science and Technology Report.
11. 1989 NHS Management Board reorganised into NHS Policy Board and NHS Management Executive.
12. 1989–1993 Establishment of NHS Trusts; Introduction of GP Fundholding.
13. 1900 New GP Contract.
14. 1990 NHS and Community Care Act introduced the Internal Market; providers of care became Trusts.
15. 1990 Family Practitioner Committees are replaced by Family Health Service Authorities; introduction of Fundholding.
16. 1991 First NHS R&D Director Appointed.
17. 1991 Research for Health Report: NHS Research Strategy published.
18. 1992 Regional R&D Directors appointed.
19. 1992 Reorganisation of Health Services in London Report.
20. 1993 Standing Committee on Health Technology Assessment established.
21. 1994 The Culyer Report; Supporting R&D.
22. 1994 Reorganisation of Regional Health Authorities.
23. 1994 Abolition of Family Health Service Authorities.
24. 1995 Regional Offices of NHS Executive established.
25. 1995 R&D Directors for Regions established.
26. 1995 House of Lords Select Committee response to The Culyer Report.
27. 1995 House of Lords Select Committee report on Academic Careers.

(Continued)

Box 4.1   (*Continued*)

28. 1997 Abolition of GP Fundholding and replaced by Primary Care Groups.
29. 2000 Abolition of NHS Executive; incorporation into the DH.
30. 2001 NHS Executive Regional Offices abolished and replaced by Regional Directorates of Health and Social care at the DH.
31. 2001 Replacement of larger health Authorities with Strategic Health Authorities.
32. 2001 Replacement of Primary Care Groups with Primary care Trusts.
33. 2002 Creation of Foundation Trusts.
34. Creation of Health and Social Care Trusts.
35. Merger of 300 Primary Care Trusts into 100 larger Trusts.
36. Merger of 28 Strategic Health Authorities into 10.
37. Reorganisation of the DH into NHS and DH.
38. 2012 Health and Social care Act 2012: Primary Care Trusts abolished and replaced by Clinical Commissioning Groups; Public Health transferred to Local Authorities.
39. 2013 Creation of NHS England with Clinical Commissioning Groups, Trust Development Authorities and Health and Health Education.

---

the service was run. It began the drive for management efficiencies in the form of targets which took little or no account of research needs. The report on medical staffing, "Hospital Staffing: Achieving a Balance" published in 1987, limited medical trainee numbers in line with clinical consultant needs, but without adequate consideration of the needs of medical research.[49] By the mid-1980s there was increasing concern that medical research was in decline as indicated by falling investment, rates of publications and citation indices[50] as well as recruitment of research trainees and clinical academics.[51] Clinical academic staff numbers fell by 12.5% between 1981 and 1987[52] and morale was reported to be in a state of collapse.[53] Among the health services research community there was also concern that dissemination of medical research findings was too slow in being reflected in clinical practice and policy making, while others felt that the focus on basic research particularly molecular biology was marginalising clinical research.[54]

House of Lords Select Committee on Science and Technology

These concerns led to the House of Lords committee on Science and Technology to undertake a review of the state of medical research in 1988.[55] This would become the most important event in transforming the prospects for health services research in recent decades and ultimately in advancing the EBM movement. The outcome of the enquiry was both remarkable and unexpected. The main reason for the enquiry had been the decline in academic medicine and yet the committee had little to say about reversing this and chose instead to make its principal recommendation the promotion of health services research, to the surprise of many.[64] To understand how this came about the deliberations of the committee are worth considering in some detail. The committee took evidence from a very wide range of bodies, was well informed and did acknowledge the depressed state of medical research in the UK. Its summary quoted from evidence given by Sir David Weatheral "British academic medicine is currently facing particularly serious problems and seems to have lost direction. There are many reasons. It has been hit hard by cuts in health service funding with deterioration in the quality of the teaching hospitals. It has also suffered from the cuts of university funding and in the availability of support from the research councils ... I hope I am not painting too gloomy a picture of the current state of medical research in the universities. I have tried to emphasise what is good, in particular the principle of the dual support system and the interaction of the government and charitable organisations in the support of research. But I hope that I have left the Committee in no doubt about the organisational problems that exist ... It is a great shame that we are facing this crisis at a time when the basic sciences are offering us the possibility of making the next 50 years the most exciting and productive for medical research; we must not miss this opportunity" (p. 25).[55]

In considering the needs of medical research, the committee accepted that "biomedical research should be science led" (p. 26)[55] and although it had some reservations that research funded by the MRC may have favoured basic research over clinical research the committee was swayed by the MRC's funding of the clinical research centre at Northwick Park, which it assumed would continue. Its conclusions in essence were to support and rely on the *status quo* to support clinical research and in doing so set aside the concerns raised by many who gave evidence. It recommended that: "(i) the present dual support systems for medical research are sound in principle, (ii) the MRC is the right vehicle for funding basic and academic clinical research and (iii) the University Grants Committee should retain responsibility for funding adequately the academic infrastructure for medical research." The committee placed the burden of supporting medical research including clinical research in the hands of the MRC on the basis of the funds returned to it from the DHSS in the concordat of 1981 and must "counter any tendency to concentrate too much on basic research when funds are short". This was in effect a continuation of the existing arrangements and was a remarkable outcome; medical research had already been in serious decline under them and so it should have been obvious that without significant changes it would continue to do so, as indeed it did.

The Committee was much more impressed by the evidence it received about the need for health services research from representatives of health economics, social medicine and the NHS Health authorities (pp. 17, 31).[55] The main deficiency it identified was a lack of NHS involvement in research. In particular it concluded that the NHS needed to identify its research needs and increase its contribution to meeting those needs. It also stressed the need to ensure that advances in research were efficiently translated into practical benefits to support the health service. "The problems" as the committee saw it "were the same failings that the Rothschild's report sought to correct in enunciating the customer–contractor principle. The NHS is the main customer for research results and so it should commission research for which it perceives a need." In effect, the committee proposed to re-enact Rothschild, but without repeating the contentious funds transfer from the MRC. The latter would continue to support medical research independently while the NHS would take primary responsibility for applied and operational research (p. 31).[56]

National Health Research Authority (NHRA)

The primary recommendation then was to bring the NHS into a central role in medical research. To achieve this, the committee proposed the establishment of a new special health authority, the NHRA. In setting out the funding role of the NHRA, the committee recommended that it should not pay for basic research, which was to remain the function of the MRC and it saw no serious overlap between the two. "The NHRA would be concerned with an applied science base which matches the service needs of the NHS. In pursuance of this end the NHRA should take on a primary role in funding public health and operational research." The NHRA would have a part role (shared with the MRC) in funding clinical research. The committee considered that the MRC "will naturally sponsor clinical research arising out of advances in science, while the NHRA will sponsor clinical research with the purpose of ensuring the development of effective new treatments and its swift transfer into service". In summarising its views, the committee envisaged two approaches to medical research; it "advocated a science-led approach in circumstances which allow research to thrive. This demands well-found laboratories, good medical schools and a strongly motivated and adequately supported body of researchers. They also recommend better recognition of the service needs of the NHS. The onus here is mainly on the NHS itself, to articulate its needs and to assist in meeting them. These two approaches — science led research and service need — then have to be welded together, so that service needs stimulate research and promising ideas flourish. Provided that successful research is then carried through into practice, these measures should have an important impact on the efficiency and cost-effectiveness of the NHS, and of national research spending, in line with the Government's overall policy." The result therefore was not so much to put the NHS into the centre of medical research, but rather to put health services research and operational research into the centre of the NHS, and the primary means to meet its service and policy needs. Basic research would be left more or less as it was, mainly funded by the MRC and clinical research would have to rely on the committee's encouragement of the MRC "to strengthen the contribution of clinicians to its work".

The Rise of Health Services Research

The outcome of the 1988 House of Lords report was a surprise to many including some health services researchers.[64] Having set out to resolve problems facing medical research it had little to say about how to resolve them other than to make the best use of what was available and instead came up with a plan to establish health services research at the centre of the NHS.

Possible reasons for this unexpected result may have included the very poor representation of medical research among the committee members. There were two advisors to the committee. Professor Walter Holland was an active leading senior member of the health service research community, he was chairman of the Directors of Health Services Research Units with close links to interests in the DHSS, which had long sought to establish it. The second advisor was also sympathetic to health services research. In particular, the committee appears to have relied heavily on Professor Walter Holland's contacts in the US during its visit there to collect evidence on the state of medical research.[56] Professor Holland had long standing contacts there in the fields of public health and health services research over many decades (pp. 97–98),[3] which may perhaps have skewed the information presented to the committee. In addition, AIDs was a relatively new and deeply worrying problem confronting health services worldwide and would have been drawn powerfully to the committee's attention as a public health challenge by a paper presented from the School of Public Health at the University of Los Angeles and California. It has also been suggested that the medical profession itself was weak in making a case in support of medical research and that it appeared to be less interested in research.[57] This does seem to have been the case to some extent. It should be remembered, however, that those responsible for the delivery of care would have been in a state of almost continuous turmoil during this period as a result of the magnitude and extent of the reforms and reorganisations (see Box 4.1) which had been taking place in the health service. This would have been a major distraction for those in the profession involved in delivering care. Nevertheless, there can be no doubt whatever about the strength of the evidence presented to the committee regarding the difficulties facing medical research. The committee's report did little to resolve them with the result that, it would continue to decline in the following years.

The reasons for this can be found in a failure to recognise the crucial role which the NHS must play in supporting clinical research and academic medicine. The concept of science led by scientists was supported, but limited to medical research funded by the MRC, which the committee saw as the main agency for supporting medical research. The MRC was urged to strengthen the role of clinicians in biomedical science, but this was far too little to address the problem. The proposed new National Health Research Authority was to focus on health services research and operational research.

Together, these two left clinical research relatively unsupported, caught between two stools. The MRC could never provide the clinical facilities needed to support clinical research and the new mandate for the NHS gave it free reign to push forward its long cherished objective to promote health services research. Just as it had been realised back in the 1920s, clinical research can only flourish in a clinical setting and with the enthusiastic support of the health service. It was a recipe which would leave clinical research in a state of continuing decline, as those who expressed reservations about it at the time feared it would.[57,58]

In contrast, health services research was set to develop rapidly. The government's response welcomed the House of Lord's report, however, it rejected the idea of the   National Health Research Authority, preferring instead to establish a Director of Research and Development[59] within the NHS, but with limited powers. However, the government did agree after further argument from the House of Lords Committee to upgrade the new post to allow him/her to be a member of the NHS Executive Board, Figure 4.1. The government also made two further stipulations; the new director should be a doctor in an effort to ensure that clinical research was not neglected, and would carry responsibility for the long established Department of Health research programme as well as the new NHS one. This left the health services research community unhappy, fearing dilution of effort and funding for advancing public health and operational research.[60] Despite these concerns, health services research would become the main focus of the new NHS R&D programme.

The NHS R&D Programme and the Founding of EBM in the UK

The first Director of R&D (DR&D) was appointed in 1991 and set about establishing a nationwide organisational structure. It was clear from the outset that the programme would be focused on applied evaluative research aimed at improving cost effectiveness and responsiveness of the service.[61] The programme would focus on health service research putting "emphasis on evaluations of the quality, effectiveness and cost of methods of disease prevention and treatment, and on research into the delivery and content of health care" and "to see good, relevant research findings made use of by NHS

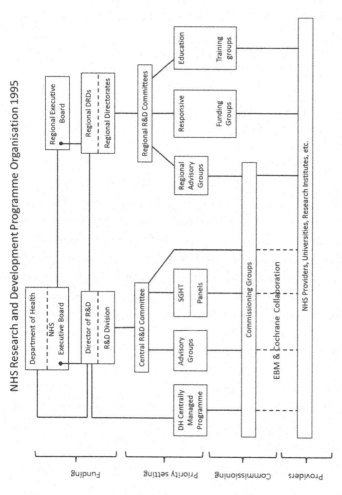

Figure 4.1   Management structure of the initial funding programme developed by the NHS director of R&D.

Note: The new R&D Director had a seat on the NHS executive and was supported by a central R&D committee in setting priorities. Except for a small centrally managed programme, almost all identified priorities were allocated to individual regional directors of R&D (DRD) for commissioning. This reflected the historical distribution of NHS support for research. The central R&D committee was supported by a number of advisory groups and a Standing Group on Health Technology (SGHT). The EBM movement was recognised early as a means to further the aims of NHS R&D and was funded by setting up a unit at Oxford and through the Cochrane Collaboration.

clinicians and managers". To achieve this, a budget of 1.5% of the total NHS budget would be sought and importantly this would include the sums already in place to support teaching hospitals to maintain their research infrastructure. However, most of these funds were already allocated to the regions and would remain so, and therefore most the R&D implementation programme would have to be devolved to the regions. A large organisational infrastructure, Figure 4.1, was also needed to manage the programme. A Central R&D committee was established to advise the DR&D in setting priorities based on political, professional, social and geographical interests and in catagorising them in order of importance; national priorities were to be funded from a limited central budget and those of national importance would be funded through the NHS regions. Each region set up its own R&D director (Regional DRD) and staff and each area of priority that had been identified was allocated to a region to take the lead on it.[62]

Once priorities were agreed, an advisory group was established for each. In addition, a Standing Group on Health Technology (SGHT) assessment was established with six panels to advise on methodologies, acute health care, diagnostics, community and primary care, drugs and screening. Each group and panel was tasked to consult widely in order to identify research needs. Recommendations were fed back to the Central R&D Committee and a commissioning group was set up for those approved, which took on the task of inviting bids from the research community, arranging external peer review and deciding whether or not to recommend funding.[63] In the years that followed, the programme and its structure altered to reflect changes to the way the NHS was managed, for example the number of regions was reduced and they were bound more closely to the NHS executive, but the research programme remained largely unchanged. A total of 5,920 applications were received between 1992 and 1995 of which 385 were funded.[64] Of these, around 100 were for systematic reviews of previously published research and marked the emphasis of comparative research to make the best use of what was known, an early example of EBM.

EBM

The new DR&D recognised information transfer between research and clinical practice as an important priority for the new programme early on.[61] At this time also, the idea of EBM was being advocated by a group of epidemiologists at McMaster University as discussed in Chapter 1 and work that would lead to the Cochrane Collaboration had also begun at Oxford. Both were almost immediately seen to be closely aligned to the priorities of the R&D programme. As a result, one of the promoters of EBM at McMaster was recruited by the Regional R&D director for Anglia and Oxford to lead a new centre of EBM based in Oxford in 1994 (pp. 65, 195)[2] and support for founding the Cochrane Collaboration was also provided. The focus on dissemination of information was also reflected in the emphasis on systematic reviews among the grants awarded by the programme. Thus, although the concept of EBM was initially marketed at McMaster University in Canada its development was to a large degree promoted in the UK as a result of the way health and science policy had evolved there. The UK NHS was the largest single provider of health care in the world and it had particular reasons to be concerned with improving cost effectiveness. Great strides had been made in increasing life expectancy and costs had risen as treatments advanced. The new challenge was to be able to fund the expanding service. This had led to a change of focus from science driven research to one of needs focused research. The timing and alignment with the emergence of EBM were perfect. The fortunes of EBM improved further with the establishment of the National Institute for Health Research (NIHR) in 2006. Infrastructural funding of clinical research in the NHS had long been provided by special allocations to teaching hospitals in recognition of the added costs required to host research. However, this had been done with little accountability. The new NIHR redistributed these funds on a competitive basis to provide infrastructural support. NIHR also established 12 large research centres as well as many research units and clinical research centres as part of a series of initiatives to reinvigorate biomedical science,[64,65] see Box 4.2. Most of these would have received funding under the previous arrangements, however, the new system ring-fenced them to avoid their diversion for general use by cash strapped hospital managers, which was an important advance. Some concentration of resources would have been achieved; however, it is difficult to determine the extent of real change or its impact. EBM continued to be strongly supported by the NIHR; by 2014, it was providing support for 20 Cochrane review groups in the UK and sponsored approximately half of all Cochrane systematic reviews undertaken.[67]

Box 4.2   NHS NIHR Initiatives 2006–2010.

1. Established Biomedical Research Centres and Units as collaborations between the NHS and medical schools.
2. Set up Clinical Research Networks.
3. Provided programme grants for applied health research.
4. Established a NIHR Faculty for all professionals and scientists engaged in applied health research or in biomedical science.
5. Offers research training awards.
6. Expanded the Health Technology Assessment (HTA) programme.
7. Set up the Public Health Research Programme to evaluate the effectiveness, cost-effectiveness and broader impact of public health interventions.

Medical Research

The House of Lords Committee on Science and Technology report of 1988 is often described as having being welcomed,[64] but a close reading of published commentaries on it[58,59,61] reveals many reservations and these were well justified in relation to the future of original medical research. Although health related research as initially envisaged by the NHS R&D directorate can be described as medical research, most of it concerned the evaluation of established knowledge to identify what is best and might be called comparative research. This is quite different from original clinical science that seeks to explore and discover new knowledge. Conflation of these two has been a consistent misconception in discussions of medical research in recent years. The new NHS directorate was happy for basic science supported by the MRC to be science-led and would encourage scientists engaged in it "to follow their instincts". However, it would not directly support curiosity driven science, but instead would focus on solving problems facing health service delivery and NHS policy needs. Implementing discoveries in basic science for the benefit of patients was regarded as a high priority and was seen as a function complementary to basic science. However, this was a profound change from how it had been supported in the past when clinical and basic research was integrated in a way that promoted a two way interaction between the clinicians and basic scientists, and facilitated the translation of discoveries in biology into clinical benefits. Crucially, the new system left clinical research to fall between the policy cracks; it could never be supported fully by the MRC alone and it was de-prioritised in the NHS R&D programme. The NHS R&D programme went further; by deciding not to directly support science led research, it in effect denied that original science was an essential component of clinical research. Added to this, the introduction of market forces to the NHS in 1992–1993 put new pressures on staff time and resources needed to conduct research and training. In response to this, The Culyer report was commissioned in 1994. This put funding for the NHS R&D programme on a more independent basis by basing it on a levy on purchasers.[68] Initially, it did little to alter the strategy of the NHS R&D programme so that the pressures on clinical researchers and their career development continued.[69] Even the NHS R&D directorate itself recognised that clinical research was still poorly supported as late as 2006[70] and these concerns remained in 2009.[71] The establishment of the NIHR in 2006 began the process of restoring an integrated approach to biomedical science by recognising the need to protect the NHS science infrastructure and ring fencing it as discussed above. Major challenges to the clinical component of biomedical science remain to be tackled. Clinical training requirements lack the flexibility needed to allow young clinicians to opt for research training with confidence for fear that their future career path will be hindered, and as a result recruitment to academic medicine is poor. NHS management targets are still too narrowly focused on limited measures of service performance; the potential value of the NHS contribution to biomedical science is immense, and needs to be recognised as a core value within the NHS executive and the DH. The NIHR is a step towards this.

Conclusions

The history of EBM is closely linked to the evolution of science policy in the UK. Although it ostensibly originated from several groups, most notably at McMaster University, it was taken up and developed predominantly in the UK, backed by the NHS. Its fortunes are linked to a debate extending back more than a century about the best way to conduct science, and how it can best meet the needs of society. The concept of science led by scientists and free from administrative interference has long been regarded as the most effective way to conduct science that explores new knowledge. That view was opposed by the idea that the primary purpose of science should be to meet the overall needs of society and therefore should be responsive to those needs. This together with the need of governments for research to assist policy making challenged the principle of scientific freedom and led to the introduction of the customer–contractor approach whereby research would be commissioned by its funders. This debate remains unresolved and both elements are in use in different sectors of research.

In the second half of the 20th century, advances in medical diagnosis and treatments contributed to major increases in health service costs. This in turn focused attention on the need for greater efficiency and cost-effectiveness. As a result, research into the way health services are organised, managed and function became important. Known as health services research, this was closely aligned with the kind of research which government departments had long sought to develop to assist policy making. For this reason, it became an important aspect of the debate between the relative values of independent science led by scientists and research commissioned for administrative and management purposes.

After an initial failure to introduce the customer–contractor principle for managing medical science in the 1970s, the House of Lords Committee of 1988 re-enacted a limited version of it within the NHS in the form of a R&D directorate which was established in 1991. This coincided with the launch of the concept of EBM, which was immediately seen as a potential new way to promote its objectives by the newly created NHS R&D directorate. With its newly acquired funds, the NHS directorate acted quickly to support the venture, initially hiring one of the founders to set up a unit of EBM in Oxford and later by funding almost half of all systematic reviews undertaken by the Cochrane Collaboration.

As EBM and other forms of health services research expanded, clinical science declined due to intense service pressure and failure to recruit young clinicians to academic careers. As EBM becomes an established aspect of medicine, so too the distinction between comparative research on which it depends and original clinical science is increasingly recognised. These prompted the establishment of the National Institute for Health Research in 2006 which successfully ring-fenced NHS support for biomedical science infrastructure. This is a first step in restoring medical research; the next must be the setting of research including original biomedical science at the core of the NHS mission. This is essential to ensure that clinical science is supported and that clinical scientists are able to provide the vital two way interaction with basic science that is needed to realise the full potential of biomedical science.

References

1. Shergold M, Grant J (2008). Freedom and Need: The Evolution of Public Strategy for Biomedical and Health Research in England. *Health Research Policy and Systems*, 6, 2.
2. Kogan M, Henkel M, Hanney S. (2006). Government and Research; Thirty Years of *Evolution*, Netherlands: Springer.
3. Holland W (2013). Improving Health Services; Background, Methods and Applications. *2013, Edward Elgar Cheltenham UK*, 61.
4. Ministry of Reconstruction (1918). Report of the Machinery of Government Committee. *HMSO*.
5. Edgerton S (2009). The Haldane principal and other invented traditions in science policy. Available at: http://www.historyandpolicy.org/policy-papers/papers/the-haldane-principle-and-other-invented-traditions-in-science-policy (Accessed on 4/12/2015)
6. (1919). *Ministry of Reconstruction: Memorandum on the Future Organisation of Medical Research*, London: HSMO.
7. Kholer RE (1978). Walter Fletcher and FG Hopkins and the Dunn Institute of Biochemistry: A Case Study of the Patronage of Science. *Isis*, 69, 331–355.
8. Austoker J (1989). *Walter Morley Fletcher and the Origins of a Basic Biomedical Research Policy. In*: Historical perspectives on the role of the Medical Research Council, (Eds). Austoker J, Bryder L. London: Oxford University Press, pp. 23–33.
9. WB (1923). The Problem of Cancer. *Natue*, 112, 101–102.
10. Research in relation to public health [lecture to the Public Health Congress 1928] pp. 41–60 and The scope and needs of medical research [lecture to the Royal Institution 1932]. Contemporary Medical Archive Centre CMAC PP/WMF/5.
11. Booth CC. *Clinical Research. In*: Histolical Perspectives on the Role of the MRC. (Eds). Austoker J, Bryder L. London: Oxford University Press, pp. 205–241.
12. Report of the Royal Commission on University Education in London (1913). London: HMSO.
13. Landsborough Thomson A (1973). *Half a Century of Medical Research*, Vol. 1, The Origins and Policy of the Medical Research Council (UK), London: HMSO.

14. Meakins JC, Parkinson J, Gunson EB, Cotton TF, Slade JG, Drury AN, Lewis T (1916). Heart Affections in Soldiers with Special Reference to Prognosis of Irritable Heart. *BMJ*, 2(2980), 418–420.

15. Lewis T (1930). Observations on Research in Medicine: Its Position and Its Needs. *BMJ*, 1(3610), 479–483.

16. Moynihan Surgery in the Immediate Future. *BMJ*, 1930(ii), 612–614.

17. Sheridan DJ (2013). Medical Science in the 21st century: Sunset or New Dawn. London: Imperial College Press, 2013.

18. Clinical Research and the Health Service. *BMJ*, 1953, July 18th (ii) 140–141.

19. Clinical Research and the Health Service. *BMJ*, 1953, July 18th (ii) 147.

20. Clinical Research in Britain 1950–1980. *In*. Wellcome Witness to Twentieth Century Medicine. Volume 7, 2000. Available at: http://www.histmodbiomed.org/sites/default/files/44829.pdf (Accessed on 4/12/2015).

21. Dr Sheila Howarth In Clinical Research in Britain 1950–1980. Wellcome witness to Twentieth Century Medicine. 2000, Vol 7, p. 10. Available at: http://www.histmodbiomed.org/sites/default/files/44829.pdf (Accessed on 4/12/2015).

22. Ford ES, Umed, Ajani A, Croft JB, Critchley JA, Labarthe DR, Kottke TE, Giles WH, Capewell S (2007). Explaining the Decrease in U.S. Deaths from Coronary Disease, 1980–2000. *N Engl J Med*, 356, 2388–2398.

23. Portfolio for Health (1971). (Ed). Mc Lachlan, Gordon 1971. London: Oxford University Press.

24. Challenges for change; *Essays on the Next Decade in the National Health Service*. (Ed). McLachlan, Gordon 1971, London: Oxford University Press.

25. Portfolio for Health. (Ed). McLachlan G, 1973. London: Oxford University Press.

26. Cohen RHL (1971). *The Departments Role in Research and Development. In*. Portfolio for Health. (Ed). Mc Lachlan G, London: Oxford University Press.

27. Modle J (1973). *Coronary Heart Disease. In*. Portfolio for Health. (Ed). Mc Lachlan G, London: Oxford University Press, pp. 71–77.

28. Cochrane A (1972). *Effectiveness and Efficiency: Random Reflections on Health Services. London*: Nuffield Provincial Trust.

29. Gabbey J, Walley T (2006). Introducing New Health Interventions. *BMJ*, 332, 64–65.

30. Committee of Enquiry into the Organisation of Civil Science (1963). *Report of the Committee of Enquiry into the Organisation of Civil Science, under the chairmanship of Sir Burke Trend.* London: HMSO.

31. Heyworth (1965). *Report of the Committee 011 Social Studies.* London: HMSO.

32. The Organisation and Management of Governement R&D by Lord Rothschild Head of the Central Policy Review Staff (1971). In A Framework for Government Research and development. London: HMSO.

33. The Future of the Research Council System (1971). *A Report of a C.S.P Working Group under the Chairmanship of Sir Frederick Dainton. In*: A Framework for Government Research and development. London: HMSO.
34. Cabinet Office (1972). *Framework for Government Research and Development. Presented to Parliament by the Lord Privy Seal by Command of Her Majesty.* London: HMSO.
35. Lord Rothschild in the Dock. *Nature*, 1972, 235, 240–240.
36. Criticisms of Rothschild Reiterated. *Nature*, 1972, 236, 50–51.
37. Dainton Demands a Hearing. *Nature* 1972, 235, 296–297.
38. Shadow of Rothschild over Strathclyde. *Nature*, 1972, 235, 71–73.
39. Rothschild's Recipe in the United States. *Nature*, 1971, 235, 301–302.
40. The Rothschild ship comes home. *Nature* 1972, 238, 124–125.
41. Gray J. *In*: Clinical Research in Britain 1950–1980. Wellcome Witness to Twentieth Century Medicine, p. 49.
42. Nairne P. *In*: Clinical Research in Britain 1950–1980. Wellcome Witness to Twentieth Century Medicine, pp. 50–51.
43. Black D AK, Pole JD (1975). Priorities in Biomedical Research: Indices of Burden. *Br J Preventive and Social Medicine*, 29, 222–227.
44. Buller A. *In*: Clinical Research in Britain 1950–1980. Wellcome Witness to Twentieth Century Medicine, pp. 56–57.
45. House of Commons, Public Accounts Committee (1979). First Report, Session 1979–80, The Ministry of Agriculture, Fisheries and Food, Department of Industry, Scottish Economic Planning Department, Welsh Office, Department of Education and Science, Medical Research Council, Scottish Home and Health Department, Agricultural Research Council, Department of Agriculture and Fisheries for Scotland. London: HMSO.
46. Beating a Retreat from Rothschild. *Nature*, 1981, 289, 2.
47. Buller A, Gowans JL (1981) Medical Research and the Funding of the MRC. *BMJ*, 282, 820.
48. Taylor D, Teeling Smiith G (1984). Health Services. *In*. UK Science Policy, A Critical review of Policies for publicly funded research. (Ed). Goldsmith Longman M London: New York.
49. Department of Health and Social Security, Joint Consultants' Committee, Chairmen of Regional Health Authorities (1987). Hospital Medical Staffing: Achieving a Balance. London: DHSS.
50. Smith R (1888). International Comparisons of Funding and Output Research: Bye Britain. *BMJ*, 296, 409–412.
51. Booth CC (1988). The National Health Service, the Universities, and the Research Councils: The Future of Academic Medicine. *BMJ*, 296, 1382–1385.

52. Cuts Force UK Universities into "Glamorous" Medical Research. *Nature*, 1987, 327, 262.
53. Medical Professors Public Complaint. *Nature*, 1987, 327, 180.
54. Smith R (1988). From the Royal Society's Meeting on the Funding of science. *BMJ*, 297, 1151.
55. House of Lords Select Committee on Science and Technology (1987–1988). Priorities in Medical research. 3rd Report session. London: HMSO.
56. Hansard HL (1988). Medical Research Priorities. Available at: http://hansard. millbanksystems.com/lords/1988/jun/15/medical-research-priorities. Vol. 498, pp. 273–245.
57. Smith R (1988). The Sickening of Medical Research: Multiple Diagnoses and Two Remedies. *Br Med J*, 296, 1079–1080.
58. Medical Research in the UK: Their Lordships View. *Lancet*, 1988, 331, 862–864.
59. Priorities in Medical Research (1990). *Government Response to the Third Report of the House of Lords Select Committee on Science and Technology: 1987–88.* London: HMSO.
60. Priorities in Medical Research. *Lancet*, 1990, 335, 284.
61. Peckham M (1991). Research and Development for the National Health Service. *Lancet*, 338, 367–371.
62. Smith R (1993). Filling the Lacuna Between Research and Practice: An Interview with Michael Peckham. *BMJ*, 307, 1403.
63. Wisely J. Haines A (1995). Commissioning a National Program of Research and Development on the Interface Between Primary and Secondary Care. *BMJ*, 311, 1080–1082.
64. Black N (1997). A national Strategy for Research and Development: Lessons from England. *Annu Rev Public Health*, 18, 485–505.
65. Department of Health (2008). Transforming Health Research. The First Two Years. National Institute for Health Progress report 2006–2008. Available at: http://www.moorfields.nhs.uk/sites/default/files/Transforming%20Health%20 Research.pdf (Accessed on 4/12/2015).
66. Department of Health (2011). National Institute for Health Research Annual report 2010/11. Available at: https://www.gov.uk/government/uploads/system/ uploads/attachment_data/file/215416/dh_130371.pdf (Accessed on 4/12/2015).
67. Bunn F, Trivedi D, Alderson P, Hamilton L, Martin A, Iliffe S (2014). The Impact of Cochrane Systematic Reviews: A Mixed Method Evaluation of Outputs from Cochrane Review Groups supported by the UK National Institute for Health Research. *Syst Rev*, 3(1), 125.

68. Culyer AJ (1994). *Supporting Research and Development in the National Health Service: A Report to the Minister for Health by a Research and Development Task Force Chaired by Professor Anthony Culyer.* London: HMSO.

69. Medical Research and the NHS Reforms: Select Committee Report. HL Deb 05 December 1995 vol. 567 cc 899–900.

70. Best Research for Best Health: A new national health research strategy. Department of Health, 2006, London: Available at: https://www.gov.uk/government/uploads/system/uploads/attachment_data/file/136578/dh_4127152.pdf (Accessed on 6/11/2014)

71. Royal College of Physicians (2009). *Innovating for Health: Patients, Physicians, the Pharmaceutical Industry and the NHS.* London: Royal College of Physicians.

Chapter 5

Hypothesis, Evidence, Knowledge and Reasoning in Medicine: Certainty and Uncertainty

"If a man will begin with certainties, he shall end in doubts"

Francis Bacon

In medicine as in all other aspects of life there are no reliable certainties in the absolute sense. In our daily lives, we draw conclusions such as "it is safe to cross the road because I see no cars coming" and we act on this with confidence. Philosophers would argue this is not a certainty pointing out the limitations of perception and reason. How can we be sure, for example, that what we see is true and not a hallucination? But it does introduce the idea of degrees of certainty or probabilities of truth. In reality, we are constantly making decisions that are based on our perceived degrees of certainty about things in order to function normally. When I say "it is safe to cross the road", I really mean that I feel certain to a sufficiently high degree, that I am willing to risk my life on it. On most occasions, we make these decisions almost unconsciously, having learned through experience how to evaluate the degree of certainty of our perception of risk and our estimate of the consequences that may follow from our decision. Indeed, it would be impossible for us to lead normal lives if we needed to evaluate every decision at a high level of consciousness. On the other hand, if the road in question is a busy one and traffic is moving fast we find ourselves acting at a much higher level of awareness in evaluating the risk, and in deciding if and when to step out. Alternatively, we may be unable to arrive at a sufficient level of certainty about the risk involved or we may judge the risk to be higher than the circumstance warrants; either would result in a retreat from the challenge. As humans, we make such decisions based on the consequences we think are likely to follow from them. Most of our decisions relate to routine activities in our lives that involve only minor consequences and we may be hardly aware we are making them; others may have major consequences for our future well-being and survival. All of our decisions require us to evaluate possible future events in this way. We begin with varying degrees of uncertainty based on our past knowledge and experience. For example, in the situation described we may already have a good idea of the likely risks based on our understanding of the road conditions, the likely volume and speed of traffic at that time of day and how the traffic is regulated at that location. You could say that we may *hypothesise* that the risk is low based on our knowledge and past experience. We would then examine the situation using the "stop, look and listen" rules learned as children to gather *evidence* about the precise conditions at the time in order to maximise our *knowledge* of the circumstances that relate to the decision we are about to make. Another way of describing this would be to say we are using our ability to reason to reduce our level of *uncertainty* about possible risks, acknowledging as Bacon expressed it in the quotation above that real *certainty* is never attainable. Humans have evolved this reasoning ability to a greater degree than all other species, and it has been the most powerful element of our survival toolkit.

Medical decision making involves highly specialised knowledge and methods of evidence gathering; however, the reasoning processes are the same; developing hypotheses, acquiring knowledge and evidence with the aim of reducing uncertainty. The beginning of any meeting between a clinician and a patient is characterised by uncertainty. Concern, fear and anxiety are also crucial aspects of the patient's perception of the encounter, and therefore what I am about to describe must take place in a context of empathy and respect for the patient's feelings and wishes. The patient's description of symptoms and the clinician's examination begin the process of evidence gathering aimed at making a diagnosis. Even at this early stage, hypotheses or possible diagnosis, based on this information coupled with previously acquired knowledge and experience, will be forming in the mind of the clinician, who will then tailor further investigations to reduce uncertainty, ultimately to a degree which leads to a decision regarding treatment, whether that be in the form of drugs, advice or simply reassurance. Although these reasoning processes remain unchanged, the nature and volume of evidence that needs to be considered have changed dramatically during the past century. In particular, advances in understanding of diseases, new and much improved diagnostic methods and treatments have greatly expanded the range and depth of knowledge which clinicians need to consider in caring for patients. There have also been major changes in the way many illnesses present, in particular the increasing prevalence of co-morbidity as we live longer. Patients understanding and expectations of medicine have also changed and clinicians must always be constantly aware that patients are individuals, and that their perceptions and descriptions of symptoms often vary considerably.

Evidence in Medicine

As discussed in Chapter 1, the Evidence-Based Medicine (EBM) movement was launched in an effort to facilitate better decision making in medicine. It focused specifically on the evidence contained in the published literature which needs to be considered by clinicians arguing that, better ways were needed to assist them in assessing and evaluating the increased volume of medical research being published. At the time, randomised controlled clinical trials had been recognised as the most reliable means for testing new treatments and were being widely adopted. This led the group to formulate the idea of medical evidence as a hierarchy with randomised clinical trials at the apex while other forms of evidence were of lesser value. It claimed to have evolved a new paradigm of medical practice and in doing so, its initial rhetoric appeared to denigrate other forms of evidence such as clinical experience and judgement. At one level, these claims might be seen as an unfortunate jibe at clinicians or a misunderstanding of what was intended and in any event both are positions the EBM movement has long abandoned attempting to defend. Nevertheless, they continue to underlie recurring controversies in medicine about the applicability of guidelines that advise on the management of groups of patients in meeting the needs of individual patients.[1]

Prophylactic Use of Anti-Flu Drugs Controversy

One example of this is the tension which has arisen, as I write, regarding the clinical use of the antiviral drugs in patients at risk of flu. General practitioners (GPs) were advised by Public Health England (PHE) to prescribe antiviral drugs to people at risk of flu, including their prophylactic use in asymptomatic persons in nursing homes.[2] However, GPs in one area were warned by local representatives of their medical association that there was insufficient evidence to justify their use in asymptomatic people.[3] Subsequently, GPs in the Thames Valley Area were sent a letter by local NHS England Team to reaffirm the advice given by PHE based on their interpretation of the evidence available on the use of anti-viral drugs.[4] The letter stated that the National Institute for Health and Care Excellence (NICE) had "approved the prophylactic use of antivirals when authorized by the Chief Medical Officer and that she had authorised the prophylactic use of antivirals the previous month". The letter went on to claim that advice from the Medical Defence Union had been sought which was reported as, "there would be an expectation on the part of the public and the legal profession that NICE guidance and PHE advice would be followed". The letter also stated that, "there is also an expectation defined in the General Medical Council's (GMC's) Good Medical Practice that a doctor will respond to an organisation advising on public health". Subsequently, GPs complained of being bullied by representatives of PHE and that "even the most thick skinned" of GPs would have found this letter to be threatening in its tone.[5] The British Medical Association then waded into the controversy telling GPs they cannot be compelled to prescribe antivirals and that they had a responsibility to follow their own judgement in deciding whether or not to do so, based on the evidence available and their knowledge of their individual patients.[6] Representatives of PHE and the Centre for Infectious Disease surveillance and Control then wrote to the British Medical Journal in an attempt to reinforce the interpretation of the evidence base on antivirals as set out by PHE in its advice to GPs.[7] This was contradicted the following day by a letter from the lead authors of the most recent Cochrane Review on anti-flu therapy claiming that it was inadequately referenced to any published evidence to justify its assertions. They also questioned whether as representatives of PHE they may have been involved in the decision making process and therefore had a conflict of interest.[8] The Medical Defence Union then intervened to clarify its advice about the medico legal implications in the event of doctors departing from guidelines.[9] Its advice was that "guidelines inform practice but don't dictate it. They do not replace the knowledge and skills of clinicians. Doctors are expected to be familiar with guidelines, but this does not mean they cannot depart from guidance when in the best interest of their patients. They must be prepared to explain and justify their decisions and actions in such cases".

Best Evidence in Medicine

This controversy is important not just because it impacts the lives and well-being of patients with or at risk of flu, but also because it exposes problems that arise when there are conflicts about the nature and quality of evidence that is used to make decisions in health care. What evidence is relevant and important in deciding treatment? How is this decided? Is one form of evidence more valuable than another? Are these the same for all agents involved? Is there a single uniform interpretation of the evidence available?

What evidence matters? This case makes clear that the evidence considered by each of those involved differs. At the top of the decision tree, we have the Chief Medical Officer who is reported to have authorised the prophylactic use of antiviral treatment during the current flu season. This we might reasonably assume is based on an assessment of the public health risk, NICE guidelines, systematic reviews and other published evidence. PHE acted on the Chief Medical Officers authorisation, citing the NICE guidelines, Systematic Reviews and other published evidence. The Cochrane systematic reviews are based on published trials that meet specified quality criteria. GPs rely on these same elements of evidence, but additionally they include the evidence they obtain from individual patients.

Should one form of evidence take precedent in making these decisions? In the example above, the answer to this question appears to depend on what is being decided, what information is available to the decider and the ethical position of the actor involved. The Chief Medical Officer carries a responsibility for advising government on policy matters, the public health and the quality and safety of clinical services. To this end the guidance of NICE and published literature including systematic reviews will be most important. He/she will have an understanding of the conditions facing clinicians but clearly cannot be aware of individual patient's circumstances and therefore cannot consider this form of evidence in detail. However, in simply authorising the use of antivirals the opportunity for others to take such evidence into account is left open. PHE have much the same responsibilities and relied on the same evidence but went further in recommending that antivirals be used prophylactically. When GPs objected, it reaffirmed its recommendation and implied that if GPs failed to comply with its advice they could be in breach of their professional responsibilities as set by the General Medical Council. In taking this position PHE appear to be relying on the idea that the evidence which has guided its decision carries more weight than a GP might have to consider and that its ethical position towards public health should take priority. GPs faced with individual patients are obliged to consider the evidence they obtain from each patient separately. They will have to consider, for example, whether the coexistence of other illnesses might complicate adding a new treatment or whether the person is capable to giving informed consent to a treatment which may provide no benefit for them and may even result in side effects. Unlike public health officials, clinicians have an ethical responsibility to their patients as individuals and therefore these are essential components of the evidence which they must consider. Thus, the evidence needed to make decisions in health care depends on the questions being asked. The anti-flu drug controversy resulted from a failure to recognise this, and an assumption that a single system of evidence gathering and interpretation can be applied generally.

Hierarchies of Evidence — A Failed Enterprise

In essence, this dispute can be seen as one of competing claims about the position of certain pieces of evidence in a hierarchy of validity. On the one hand, carefully done randomised controlled trials are widely acknowledged to be the most reliable way to test for benefits of new treatments and public health experts regard these most powerful. Clinicians on the other hand must add to that the evidence about each patient's condition. Both positions are justified in the context of the ethical responsibilities of each actor and each must balance the evidence available and relevant to the decision to be taken. A problem arises (i) if one actor takes the view that its ethical responsibilities take precedent or (ii) that its view of what constitutes the most valid evidence takes priority. In this case, PHE in acting to try to reduce the overall burden of flu in the community is perceived by clinicians to disregard their obligation to their individual patients. Since the ethical position of each is valid, that is, protection of public health and individual patient health are both intrinsically good, it follows that the main basis for this dispute is in the interpretation of evidence and the question, is there a hierarchy of evidence that could be applied to the decisions each is required to make? The answer to this is clearly no. First, the evidence available to clinicians and public health physicians is different and therefore neither can ever assess the full complement of evidence available to the other. Second, the questions being asked and the decisions made by each are different and therefore the evidence which each needs to assemble and prioritise differs. So each of the actors involved, had different assemblies of evidence available to them. This means that all of it could not be accommodated in a single hierarchy that each of them could evaluate. Therefore, the concept of a hierarchy of evidence that could be applied to health care as a general tool is invalid.

Evidence and Interpretation

However, in the case cited here, even the published evidence itself and the guidelines resulting from it are hotly disputed. NICE guidelines published in 2008[10] were based on evidence at that time and were not updated following a later Cochrane review published in 2014. The authors of that Cochrane review wrote to the Chairman of NICE challenging its decision not to review its guidance in light of its latest review. PHE cited the 2014 Cochrane review in relation to its recommendation to GPs, but cautioned that since it included only randomised controlled trials and thus excluded observational data, the Cochrane review did not justify a review of its policy.[2] Subsequently the Cochrane authors criticised PHE's interpretation of the evidence.[3] This debate underlines the reality that evidence is not a kind of truth but is always open to interpretation based on the knowledge, experience and potential conscious or unconscious bias of the interpreter. Indeed we should not be surprised that clinical trial data and systematic reviews are disputed as we saw in the anti-viral case and in other well publicised cases.[11] Furthermore, maintaining up to date iterations of systematic reviews is a formidable challenge and frequently not met.[12]

In many circumstances, differing interpretations of evidence are accepted as part of a discussion that leads to better understanding. In this case, the rhetoric and manner of the debate may reflect additional factors in play. There seems little disagreement that current antiviral drugs for influenza are not a major advance and most accept that the benefit — risk ratio is marginal. Yet, the UK and US Governments have reportedly spent £424 million ($609) and $1.5 billion respectively in stock piling it and have been criticised for doing so.[13] Could there be pressure to find a use for such a large investment before it is time expired? Some have implied that public health experts may have a conflict of interest in recommending it.[8] At the other end of the story there is strong evidence that GPs have felt under pressure. In part, their objection to the prophylactic use of antivirals was due to fears that they would not have the resources to do it properly. They pointed to the fact that before prescribing a drug with a marginal risk benefit ratio in well people, careful discussion and obtaining consent would be necessary and would need considerable resources. This was particularly so for elderly people in nursing homes many of whom may be confused. As one GP put it "without extra resources what work would PHE suggest that primary care staff stop doing to fit this in?".[14] In addition, seasonal flu is demanding on health services, and this was especially the period at the time this issue arose with several hospitals in crisis due to increased demand especially in accident and emergency departments. Reducing the overall burden of seasonal flu is important in mitigating demand and vaccinating risk groups against influenza plays a role in this. No doubt, it was hoped that the use of antivirals would also be helpful. It is clear that here again there is considerable pressure related to a service struggling to meet demand. Such pressures undoubtedly add to the difficulties faced by all parts of the health service and explain the tension and rhetoric used in what one commentator described as a, "toxic and dangerous environment in which to practice medicine".[6]

However, it is important that the tension and heat generated by this case does not obscure the fact that in essence this was a dispute about evidence and claims to priority based on its interpretation. This can be traced to the notion of a hierarchy of evidence in medicine and that certain forms of evidence are more powerful for deciding what is best practice. It was advocated by the EBM movement which put forward the idea that randomised clinical trials should trump clinical evidence in decision making, as discussed in Chapter 1. Although well intended to encourage medicine based on the best published evidence for treatments, it failed to recognise the importance of the ethics and evidence related to individual patient care. This may in part reflect the group's composition, which was largely of epidemiologists. The anti-flu drug case illustrates the difficulties which arise when this is applied in healthcare. Thus, even if there were such a principal as a hierarchy of evidence validity, no single hierarchy could accommodate all of the evidence that had to be considered by those involved. Experts in public health, systematic reviewers of literature and clinicians caring for individual patients have different ethical responsibilities, and must evaluate different assemblies of evidence. Under such complex circumstances, the notion of a hierarchy of evidence seems a failed enterprise.

EBM and Myth-Making Rhetoric

Although the promotion of a hierarchy of evidence in medicine was intended to enhance the reputation of randomised controlled clinical trials and comparative research, it frequently took the form of emphasising the limitations of clinical expertise and judgement, which were allocated to a lower position in the proposed hierarchy. Several arguments were put forward to suggest the limitations of clinical expertise and judgement. As discussed in Chapter 1, fictional scenarios of clinical cases in which clinical judgements and opinions of authoritative experts proved incorrect compared to literature searches were used as rhetorical support for the launch of EBM.[15,16] Several accounts of anecdotes experienced have also been published in support of it. For example, Archie Cochrane's experience in conducting a clinical trial of the utility of coronary care units is often cited in relation to this (p. 163).[1] Cochrane relates that clinicians refused to participate in the trial "because they still felt a sacred right to treat patients as they wished", and thus suggesting that clinician's reluctance to participate was because of their belief in the superiority of their clinical judgement. However, as I have pointed out in Chapter 2,

Cochrane's account of this is inaccurate. Clinicians at the time were concerned that randomisation in the trial would prove difficult for practical and clinical reasons and that it would be of limited usefulness for this reason.[17,18] They believed that conducting a trial that had little prospect of producing useful results would be unethical. Their concerns were in fact justified when the trial went ahead as only 28% of patients were randomised[19] and this fell further to 23% in a follow up study.[20] In reality, coronary care units and the clinicians who worked in them were exceptionally enthusiastic and willing participants in many clinical trials.

Cochrane's anecdote of his experience as a medical officer during WWII to imply the futility of clinical experience is also frequently cited (p. 165).[1] He recounts that he was a single handed medical officer responsible for the care of 20,000 prisoners. Despite epidemics of typhoid, diphtheria, infections, jaundice and sand-fly fever with more than 300 cases of pitting oedema above the ankles, only four died of whom three had been shot. He suggests that this "excellent result" in the absence of specific therapy demonstrates the limited value of "clinical skills". Cochrane's description of his experiences during WWII are impressive and often moving, however, he gives us no idea of how he gathered information about illness among such a large number of prisoners, or the likely accuracy of the diagnoses he describes, given the difficulties he faced as a single handed medical officer. Cochrane's passion and willingness to put himself in harm's way are impressive and may lead to some reluctance to question the accuracy of his recollections. However, the reliability of his accounts of serious illness and survival here must surely be questionable. He went on to recount how, when he asked for medical help he was told by a German officer, "No, doctors are superfluous". Although horrified at the time, he tells us that he later became convinced that this advice "was right". However, Cochrane also seems to have had a deep seated antipathy towards clinical medicine, perhaps related to his experience of a lack of sympathy when seeking help as a teenager, his unhappiness as a medical student and his admitted unsuitability to clinical medicine; it may also explain a reluctance to seek clinical help himself and to an incorrect self-diagnosis as discussed in Chapter 2. Cochrane was a passionate advocate of comparative research; however, his enthusiasm seems to have led him infrequently into myth-making rhetoric.

Clinical Judgement versus Mechanical Rules

Clinical judgement has also been suggested to be of limited value because of its failure to perform as well as "mechanical rules", adding further weight to its low ranking by the EBM movement in the proposed hierarchy of evidence. Studies demonstrating the superiority of "mechanical rules" over "clinical judgement" in diagnosis are often cited in support of this view. One often cited study compared computer assisted diagnosis with "clinical judgement" in diagnosing abdominal pain and appendicitis, and found that the computer's system produced a significantly greater diagnostic accuracy than clinicians.[21,22] The authors of the study proposed it as a possible method for assisting and improving diagnostic accuracy; however, it has been used as evidence of the superiority of "mechanical rules" over what is referred to as "clinical judgement" (p. 168).[1] In reality this study compared the computer's ability to compute a diagnosis based on the clinical features described by clinicians with the clinicians own diagnosis based on their clinical findings. The study was an interesting initial attempt to evaluate the possible role of computers to assist diagnosis. However, it had several major limitations and its findings have not been confirmed. It was not blind or randomised, the data entered for each patient was not tabulated in the results and it is unclear whether the data considered in both arms for each patient were the same. However, setting all of these problems aside, this was not a study which compared "mechanical rules" and "clinical judgement" as has been claimed (p. 168).[1] It was in reality a comparison of data interpretation by a computer system and by clinicians. All of the data considered in both arms of this study were collected by clinicians and involved exercising clinical skill and judgement. Equating clinical judgement to data interpretation in this narrow sense trivialises it. It denigrates not only clinical skills, knowledge and experience but also the human interaction which characterises medicine and illness. Furthermore, a careful reading of the study shows that the authors of the study never intended that it should be interpreted in that way.

Mechanical Rules and Public Health Screening

Another example which illustrates the consequences of discarding clinical experience and judgement in favour of rules based management is that of a nurse who returned to the UK from Sierra Leone, where she had been working in a Ebola treatment centre.[23] On her return at Heathrow airport she had been feeling feverish and unwell and was concerned about having possibly contracted Ebola. Her temperature was taken using an ear thermometer and found to be "within range" and she was allowed to proceed to her connecting flight. However, she felt more feverish one hour later and returned to the screening centre where her temperature was taken a further six times and again found to be "within range" and she was allowed onto her flight. Her condition worsened and after returning home in a taxi she was admitted to hospital and confirmed to have contracted the disease. In this case, all of the rules were followed but failed to diagnose the case correctly. It is clear that the officials applying the rules did so meticulously, indeed exhaustively having repeated taking her temperature 6 times. The "system" was said to have "worked" meaning that the rules were followed correctly as if this somehow exonerated its failure. Later, senior public health figures acknowledged that a more "precautionary approach" would have been appropriate, particularly since the nurse was due to fly again exposing many other people to the risk of infection.

The question then arises how would a "more precautionary" approach be implemented? The obvious answer is by the application of a smidgen of clinical judgement. Any health worker with clinical experience in managing cases of infectious diseases would be expected to evaluate and take into account the background travel history, and how the person was feeling in reaching a likely diagnosis.[24] But this would entail all of the reasoning processes described above; evidence gathering and hypothesis making in the context of knowledge of the condition. None of this is possible by the application of mechanical rules, which in this case involved the use of decisions made in advance without evidence or knowledge of the person's symptoms or signs, with the exception of temperature measurement. The case illustrates well the limitations of attempting to apply mechanical rules in health care. Mechanical rules may have a place in screening healthy people with an inherently very low risk as a public health measure, however, they have no place in caring for people who are actually ill and seeking medical care.

Clinicians may encounter cases in which they believe their expertise and judgement were vital in caring for a patient. Supporters of mechanical rules may argue that a comparison of such cases with rule-based systems does not stand because there was no rule available and in such a situation the sensible and "mechanical" course of action would be to "do more tests" (p. 175).[1] It raises a number of relevant questions. If no rule exists, how would a suitable rule be designed to accommodate this particular situation, given its unique characteristics; how would rules be designed to take account of the many illnesses which afflict humans and the variability in their presentation from one person to the next? The argument that the default position, "do more tests" applies in a situation where no rule exists or when a clinician faces a serious condition might seems sensible. In reality, the "do more tests" rule is almost meaningless. The problem is that "do more tests" could mean anything from taking a blood test or measuring the temperature and may be useless when a specific course of action is required. Indeed, the "do more tests" rule was the response in the Ebola case and resulted in a "do-loop" of repeated temperature measurements that were unhelpful. The operation of pre-determined mechanical rules carries the promise of efficiency and lower cost of implementation, mainly by avoiding consumption of time and expensive human reasoning that requires knowledge and experience and the ability to collect and evaluate evidence. Such techniques may have contributed to dramatic increases in industrial productivity during the 20th century, however, attempts to apply them to situations in which human experience needs to be evaluated have failed drastically as I have argued previously.[25] The immense variety of experiences that accompany illness in humans and how those experiences are expressed can only be evaluated through human interaction requiring clinical expertise and judgement. In addition, respect and empathy for the experiences of ill patients are crucial for restoring health and well-being and this too requires appropriate individual human interaction. Attempts to relegate these in favour of industrial management techniques have also caused great harms to patients and health care delivery.[26]

The corollary may also arise. A clinician might respond when pressed to follow clinical guidelines in caring for a patient that "this patient is different from those for whom clinical guidelines were written and therefore I cannot follow them". First, we should distinguish between mechanical rules and clinical guidelines. The former should be restricted to predetermined rules that do not require clinical expertise or judgement for their implementation, and have no place in clinical management. Clinical guidelines on the other hand are schedules of advice related to defined clinical conditions and require clinical knowledge, expertise and judgement in order to apply them. The anti-viral drug controversy described above and the discussion surrounding it makes clear that clinical guidelines are advisory; they are not commands or "rules". Clinicians must be aware of them and be prepared to use them. However, it is also recognised that following a clinical guideline is not an acceptable defence against harm caused to a patient if it was applied inappropriately due to some unique feature of their case. Thus clinicians must always exercise judgement in deciding to follow guidelines. By the same token should a clinician decide to depart from guidelines they must be prepared to explain and defend their clinical judgement.

Diagnostic Criteria

The Ottawa Ankle Rules system is widely used to assess the likely risk of ankle fracture and has been shown to reduce the number of unnecessary X-ray examinations.[27] It too has been claimed as support for the view that "mechanical rule following is superior to expert clinical judgement"(p. 168).[1] The case rests on the fact that when "mechanical rules" were applied to patients seen following ankle injury, fewer X-rays were ordered, reducing costs and time spent in hospital with no reduction in diagnostic accuracy or patient satisfaction.[28] But here too the argument fails for several reasons. The description of the Ottawa Ankle Rules as "mechanical" in this context is again misleading in that it implies a system that is quite separate and independent of clinical expertise or judgement; one that involves no interaction with the patient and one that might be used to replace clinical expertise and judgement. The authors of the Ottawa rules more accurately described it as "clinical decision rules", but the more generally accepted term diagnostic criteria would apply equally well. They are in fact a system based on a thorough clinical examination to determine the presence or absence of pain at defined anatomical sites on both sides of the ankle, and whether the patient can bear weight on it. A list of clinical features so identified is then used to diagnose the likelihood of a fracture. Therefore application of such rules implicitly requires the use of clinical expertise and judgement, negating the idea that they might somehow be superior to or be capable of replacing clinical expertise. What these rules really provide is a reminder for the clinician to include all of the relevant parts of the examination and a guide to their interpretation. It also provides a recognised and validated system of practice for deciding whether the patient needs an X-ray, which could be used as a defence against claims of malpractice in the event of a fracture not detected.[29] This I suggest is also significant in reducing defensive practice and the number of X-ray examinations carried out. Thus again, the implication that the usefulness of these rules indicate that they are superior to and might be used to replace clinical expertise and judgement is misleading, since the use of the rules depends on both.

Duckett Jones Diagnostic Criteria for Rheumatic Fever

The Ottawa Rules are in reality, examples of diagnostic criteria, the use of which to improve diagnostic accuracy in clinical medicine is not new. In the early years of the 20th century rheumatic fever was a major cause of ill health. Acute rheumatic fever in Western Countries most frequently occurred in childhood and was a serious illness which could be fatal. It also resulted in the delayed appearance of valvular heart disease and chronic ill health. The clinical features of rheumatic fever were often quite variable making diagnosis a challenge. They included carditis (inflammation of the heart), arthritis, chorea (a disturbance of the central nervous system), skin rash, subcutaneous nodules and pericardial rub among others. Thomas Duckett Jones began to study such cases in 1928 and over several years documented the variety of clinical presentations associated with the condition, noting for example the significance of chorea in 1935.[30] By studying the clinical details of a 1,000 patients Duckett Jones and colleagues were able to determine the incidence of symptoms and signs of the illness and thereby to assemble criteria in order of importance in diagnosing the condition.[31] Clinical diagnostic criteria such as this are not separate, independent or a sort of possible replacement for clinical expertise and judgement. They are in fact an intrinsic component of it and have been taught to medical students as such during their clinical training for several decades.

In summary, "mechanical rules" and "decision rules" are not appropriate in clinical medicine involving the care of individual patients. They imply the predetermined control of decisions which cannot take account of individual patients' clinical features. They should not be confused with clinical guidelines which are not rules, but advisory and they require clinical expertise and judgement to be applied properly. Even when guidelines may be applicable to a majority of patients seen they still need to be considered for each individually. Automatic or mechanical application of a guideline would not be defensible action if it resulted in patient harm.[9] Diagnostic criteria takes the form of list of clinical features and test results that are helpful in clarifying a diagnosis. Again, they are advisory not rules and they require clinical expertise and judgement to be applied. Clinical guidelines and diagnostic criteria are well established systems to assist best practice and both require clinical expertise and judgement to be implemented safely. It follows that comparisons of patient outcomes based on clinical judgement and clinical guidelines are specious.

The Role of Evidence in Clinical Judgement

I have stressed the importance of evidence derived from individual patients; however, evidence and knowledge derived from study, experience, and the published literature are also key elements in clinical decisions. I have also argued that different assemblies of evidence are needed to deal with challenges faced in separate parts of health care and therefore that no single hierarchy could accommodate all of them. The question remains whether a hierarchy could have utility in less complex situations, for example, to the evidence which must be considered by clinicians managing individual patients? The EBM movement argued that it can on the basis of carefully done clinical trials in adequate numbers of patients provide a more reliable method to determine best practice than "clinical judgement" or "mechanistic reasoning" as discussed in Chapter 1. In this context, clinical judgement is considered to be an intuitive guess or hunch and mechanistic reasoning is an argument in favour of a particular treatment on the basis of some known physiological or biochemical mechanisms. The rhetoric is generally one in which, clinicians are presented as protective of a right to do as they wish and resistant to undertaking clinical trials and accepting their results. Examples are then presented in which carefully done trials trump such judgements, (see p. 122).[1]

Expert Opinion and Clinical Judgement

A key article published in 1992 showed that opinions expressed in review articles about treatments over the preceding 30 years were frequently out of date, compared with cumulative systematic reviews, which provide an iterative statistical method for synthesising clinical trial data as it is published.[32] Many of the recommendations of experts did not take account of most of the recent research, some were indicated inappropriately and other treatments for which evidence of benefit were not recommended. This will not have been a great surprise to clinicians many of whom regarded "textbooks as being out of date as soon as they were written". The lead author of the study, Thomas Chalmers is justly lauded for this work, the culmination of a career devoted to developing statistical tools for synthesising the results of separate clinical trials. Chalmers established beyond doubt what many suspected in calling for more rapid and timely systematic reviews to help disseminate more accurate and reliable information. Systematic reviews, also known as meta-analyses subsequently have become widely adopted in medicine. The EBM movement was particularly active in promoting these methods and subsequently founded the Cochrane Collaboration to provide a system for producing them. So too have many other researchers and academic units.

This is powerful evidence that statistical methods are in most cases likely to be superior to an opinion about treatments and this is still likely to be true in most instances. It would of course depend to some degree on whether an up to date meta-analyses is available, and whether an opinion had taken due notice of it. If for example, an expert was fully aware of and took into account results of the most recent meta-analysis, would such an opinion be less accurate than the meta-analysis itself and which should occupy the top of a hierarchy of evidence? Putting aside other potentially confounding factors for the moment they should theoretically be of equal merit. Therefore to say that an opinion is more valid simply because it is derived from one source, (say a statistician), rather than another (say a clinician) is not justified. The Chalmers study showed that the published opinions of experts had not taken account of all of the available evidence at the time, but also pointed to the lack of efficient tools to allow them to do so. We now have thousands of systematic reviews, which are used to develop guidelines for treatment and clinicians are required to keep their knowledge of them up to date. Which of these should occupy the top of a supposed hierarchy of evidence?

The answer to this would seem to depend on what question the evidence is to be used to answer. To the question "what is the best published evidence about the use of drug A in treating condition B?", either a randomised controlled clinical trial would be the ideal or in the case where several trials have been published, a meta-analysis of them. To answer the question "what is the best and most cost effective treatment for condition B and how does drug A perform?", a review of all randomised controlled trials and meta-analyses together with as assessment of the cost effectiveness of drug A. To answer the question "Is drug A suitable for my patient and is it indicated?", knowledge of the first two is necessary, but also evidence and knowledge about the patient. It would not be appropriate for example to give an anticoagulant to prevent deep vein thrombosis to someone who has a high risk of bleeding, neither might it be appropriate to give a drug of marginal benefit to someone who is well in the hope of preventing an illness as discussed above in relation to anti-viral treatment. These are vital matters when dealing with individual patients in clinical medicine, which cannot be "trumped" by statistical evidence no matter how elegantly calculated.

Discussions about medical evidence often use the term clinical judgement to refer to different things. Comparisons of clinical trial data and expert opinions published in review articles frequently refer to the latter as clinical judgements (p. 158).[1] But they are not; they are in reality opinions about treatments from a variety of experts some of whom may be clinicians and are generally put forward on the basis of an individual reading of selected literature. As such they are highly unlikely to be as reliable as meta-analyses, but this is true irrespective of whether written by clinicians or other specialists. They are less reliable because of the methods they use to arrive at the opinions expressed; whether they are clinicians or not is irrelevant. Clinical judgement should be used to describe the use of actual observations made about a patient, together with other data to arrive at a decision. It follows that clinical judgement and comparative research are quite different things and are simply not comparable in terms of their validity. The question as to which should occupy a higher or lower position in a supposed hierarchy of evidence is not sensible. It is clear that clinical trials and meta-analyses provide the best research evidence about treatments. Both are valuable forms of evidence which clinicians must be familiar with in making decisions. There are elements of "other data" that must be considered in making clinical judgements. Thus, the concept of a hierarchy of evidence fails even when applied to decisions made in the context of a single illness involving one patient.

Although the paper by Chalmers *et al.* cited above[32] referred to inaccuracy of expert reviews compared with meta-analyses, the idea seems to have morphed into a general stereotypical view of clinical experts and figures of (clinical) authority or seniority as unreliable, promoted by the EBM movement and its advocates.[15,16,33] Conflating opinions expressed in expert review articles with clinical judgement in this way facilitated the idea of clinical judgement as less reliable in the proposed hierarchy of evidence.[16] Although the EBM movement retreated from this view,[34] it continues to linger in discussions about EBM (p. 167).[1] The idea of a hierarchy of evidence with clinical judgement in a lower tier than comparative research would in effect establish a higher authority of validity in the latter. This I suggest underlies much of the controversy which has arisen in the cases discussed above. For example, the tensions which emerged between PHE and GPs over the former's recommendation about the use of anti-viral drugs to prevent flu in healthy people are a direct consequence of such a view. The public health experts clearly believed that they had a better grasp of what they considered the relevant evidence and sought to exert authority over their GP colleagues to carry out their recommendations. But the GPs were having none of it because of their need to consider the evidence obtained from their patients individually. It follows that evidence which is derived from each patient is central to all clinical judgement. The interpretation and application of other evidence and knowledge will always be dependent on it. In the case of clinical medicine it may be better to think of primary evidence as that involving the patient, including clinical symptoms and signs, as well as the patient's fears, hopes and wishes and secondary evidence as all other data and knowledge that may serve to best care for the patient. This places the interests of patients at the heart of the care system, while ensuring that clinicians respond to their patients' best interest by taking into account all of the available evidence including research evidence, as they are professionally obliged to do. Figure 5.1(a) illustrates the original simplified concept of a hierarchy of evidence suggested by the EBM movement. The limitations of this were recognised and a modified version was put forward in 1996, Figure 5.1(b). However, this too failed to recognise the role that clinical expertise plays in gathering information from patients and in making clinical decisions. An alternative model is proposed to include Figure 5.1(c).

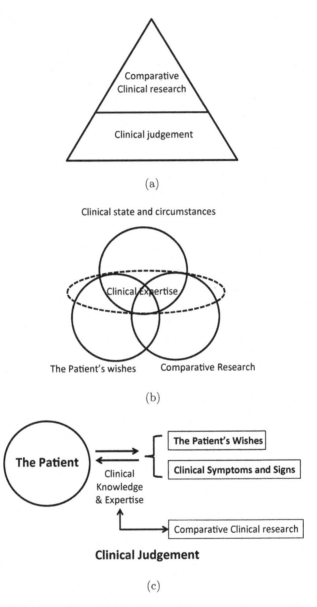

Figure 5.1   Concept of a hierarchy of evidence with comparative research at the top was advanced by the EBM movement in early 1990s (a).[15,16] In a later version this was modified (b) to acknowledge a central role of clinical expertise in implementing decisions in patient care, while taking account of the patient's wishes and clinical features as well as research evidence.[36] However, model (b) proposes clinical expertise as separate from the

---

Figure 5.1   (*Continued*) clinical state of the patient. Since evidence about the clinical state of the patient is gathered using clinical expertise, this separation would distort the process of clinical decision making. Model C is proposed to show that such decisions are made in relation to individual patients, taking account of actual evidence gathered from the patient using clinical expertise, together with other relevant data. It places patients' wishes and clinical features as of primary important and recognises the role of clinical expertise in gathering that evidence. It also acknowledges the role of clinical expertise in interpreting and applying research evidence to individual patients in making clinical judgements.

Mechanistic Reasoning and EBM

Advances in medicine have been based to a large degree on understanding mechanisms of normal and abnormal function in the body. For example, understanding the role of insulin in enabling glucose transport across cell membranes helped to advance knowledge about diabetes. Similarly the discovery that aspirin inhibits activation of platelets led to its use in preventing heart attacks in patients with coronary heart disease. Mechanistic reasoning uses general knowledge of such cause – effect relationships in order to develop theories about specific questions. Knowledge that platelet activation is involved in the development of coronary thrombosis and that aspirin inhibits platelet activation led to the theory that aspirin would prevent coronary thrombosis. This would be a typical example of mechanistic reasoning and is one form of evidence which could be considered in arriving at a clinical decision. It is of course insufficient evidence to establish efficacy of aspirin in this situation and is therefore, of limited value. It is however, powerful evidence in generating a hypothesis of efficacy, and therefore, a rational and ethical basis for testing the possibility in patients. This is necessary since the use of aspirin may also carry a risk of harm such as bleeding.

The original proposal of EBM emphasised randomised controlled trials as the most reliable evidence for clinical decisions and considered mechanistic reasoning as unreliable and possibly dangerous,[15,16] a view that has persisted. Thus, mechanistic reasoning was placed very low or not at all in ratings of evidence quality.[35] The basis for this was the publication of many clinical trials which showed clear evidence of benefit or harm contradicting theories previously held based on mechanistic reasoning. One often cited example of this is the Cardiac Arrhythmia Suppression Trial (CAST) which studied the effect of the Class 1C anti-arrhythmic drugs flecainide and encainide on mortality following myocardial infarction.[36] The trial was based on the hypothesis that many such patients died suddenly due to lethal arrhythmias and it had been shown that both drugs were capable of reducing arrhythmias in such patients. The question remained as to whether this would translate to a reduction in deaths. The trial went ahead in the US and its data monitoring committee ordered it to be stopped when it detected clear evidence of increased deaths among patients receiving either of these drugs compared with placebo.[36] These included a greater number of deaths due to arrhythmia or cardiac arrest, 33 of 730 patients in the active treatment group compared with 9 of 725 in the placebo group. Thus the hypothesis did not just fail; it was contradicted by the findings. These results have been repeatedly cited[37–39] (p. 136),[1] as evidence of the weakness of mechanistic reasoning, backed by evidence in a book published by Thomas Moore in 1995.[40] The book entitled "Deadly Medicine" with the subtitle "Why tens of thousands of heart patients died in America's worst drug disaster" printed on the front cover claimed that as many as 50,000 people died during the period in which the CAST study was recruiting patients to the trial and likened the toll to events such as the Vietnam War. However, even these claims were exaggerated further to 70,000 deaths each year in arguing the dangers of mechanistic reasoning.[35,37,39]

On the face of it this appears to be a damning result for mechanistic reasoning in clinical medicine. But is this a fair analysis? First, is it correct to assume that the hypothesis tested in the CAST study had been used to justify treating asymptomatic patients with ventricular ectopic beats following myocardial infarction with flecainide and encainide? Encainide was not available in the UK and such treatment was certainly not routine there. In the US, flecainide had been available since 1986 and encainide since 1987 and prescribing would have been possible; however, neither of these drugs were licenced for treating patients with asymptomatic ventricular arrhythmias. The dramatic claims made for the large number of deaths caused by these drugs were based on major assumptions.[40] In his analysis, Moore extrapolated the effects seen in the CAST study, to all class 1 anti-arrhythmic agents and to all patients receiving anti-arrhythmic treatment, both of which are invalid. A study of overall anti-arrhythmic drug usage and deaths from coronary heart disease in the US between 1982 and 1991 examined this question.[41] Flecainide was marketed in the US in 1986 and encainide in 1987. All Class 1C anti-arrhythmic drugs sales peaked in 1987 and 1988 and amounted to 20% of all anti-arrhythmic drug sales. Overall sales of Class 1 anti-arrhythmic drugs declined by 3% and 4% during the 2 years before CAST was published in April 1989 and more sharply thereafter by 12%. Sales of Class 1C drugs fell dramatically by 75% after CAST was published. Deaths from coronary heart disease in the US followed a continuous linear decline during 1982 to 1991 and no deviation in the linear trend was observed either upward (during 1986–1989 when Class 1C sales peaked) or downward (after 1989 when Class 1C sales plummeted). Claims of excess deaths in the range suggested by Moore were readily excluded by the 95% confidence intervals of the predicted linear trend.[41] Thus, the exaggerated claims of harm due to the use of these drugs were unfounded. This also indicates that repeated claims (p. 126)[1,35,37,39] that clinicians were prescribing class 1C antiarrhythmic drugs for this group of patients on the basis of mechanistic reasoning are incorrect.

Mechanistic Reasoning and Clinical Medicine

What role if any can mechanistic reasoning play in clinical medicine? Examples mentioned above are helpful in this respect. Considering the role of aspirin to reduce the risk of coronary thrombosis, there were mechanistic reasons to suggest its use (it was known that aspirin inhibits platelet activation[42] and that platelet activation was involved in coronary thrombosis). These however, would not have been sufficient to justify its use without further evidence. That further evidence came from controlled clinical trials.[43] Therefore, one can say that such clinical trials were vital in developing this treatment and in justifying its widespread use. However, aspirin also has important side effects including the risk of bleeding, stomach ulcers and stroke. To embark on a trial of this kind requires a hypothesis of potential benefit based on some form of evidence. That evidence involved reasoning about the mechanisms which mediate the action of aspirin and of coronary thrombosis. Thus, mechanistic reasoning provided the necessary scientific and ethical basis to justify including patients in the trial. Similarly, the CAST study design was clearly based on the hypothesis that flecainide and encainide would reduce deaths due to arrhythmias in patients following myocardial infarction having established their anti-arrhythmic potential in those patients. We can say therefore that in this study also mechanistic reasons were used to justify the study. Would these examples of mechanistic reasoning have been sufficient to justify the use of aspirin or flecainide in clinical practice? The answer here must be no and this appears to have been the way clinicians acted despite claims to the contrary. Indeed, clinicians have been considered tardy in using aspirin to treat patients with coronary disease following the publication of clinical trial evidence.[32] Thus, it seems clear that mechanistic reasoning has an important role in medical research; that includes not only original exploratory science, but also clinical trials and therefore all comparative research. Bearing in mind that maintaining and advancing knowledge are components of medical professionalism it follows that this also applies to physicians.

Should clinical judgements include mechanistic reasoning? The CAST study again offers a good example of mechanistic reasoning proving to be misleading if applied in making clinical judgements. Its fundamental weakness relates to incomplete knowledge. Understanding of a cause effect relationship related to a particular mechanism cannot be extrapolated safely to complex biological systems. For example, if our knowledge of the regulation of the heart rhythm is incomplete then a hypotheses based on a particular part of it may fail if applied to the whole, due to unforeseen interactions. This is a good reason for caution in mechanical reasoning and especially so in relation to decisions that carry potential risks for patients. It has been a feature of the EBM movement to pitch its case on the basis of an all or none comparison of comparative research and mechanistic reasoning and presenting the latter as dangerous and unreliable. But this is an over simplistic view. Notwithstanding the availability of a mechanistic reason for using Class 1C anti-arrhythmic agents, clinicians may already have been showing such caution about them; clinicians had already begun to observe and publish case reports of their possible pro-arrhythmic effects [44,45] and their use had already been in decline prior to the publication of CAST.[41] This suggests that physicians are not necessarily waylaid by such reasoning, but open to other sources of knowledge and information. Furthermore, clinicians face daily questions about the applicability of recommendations, guidelines and research evidence to their individual patients and making such decisions inevitably involves elements of mechanistic reasoning. This has been acknowledged more formerly in philosophical terms[46]; physicians know it from experience and argue that it is essential in recognising patients as individuals with unique experiences.[47] Thus, mechanistic reasoning is unavoidable in medicine and plays an important role in managing uncertainties which arise in clinical practice and in applying research evidence to individual patients. In situations where no research evidence is available, mechanistic reasoning may in fact dominate management. Recently in a small number of cases of Ebola infection, patients were given antibodies collected from previously infected patients who had survived, based on the hypothesis that they would help to clear the virus by destroying it. In the absence of trial data, this is based entirely on mechanistic reasoning and has not received any serious criticism. However, to rely on such evidence solely when good research evidence is available would be unprofessional. On the other hand, to exclude the use of mechanistic reasoning entirely would reduce medicine to a level of mechanical rules and deny the individuality of patients.

Conclusions

Hypothesis making, evidence gathering, knowledge and reasoning are all essential and unavoidable elements of the process of caring for patients. Research evidence from clinical trials and comparative research were introduced on a large scale during the 20th century to establish evidence of efficacy and harm of new treatments and are an essential component of the evidence which needs to be considered in making clinical decisions and judgements.

The concept of a hierarchy of evidence proposed by the EBM movement suggested that medical evidence could be arranged and evaluated such that comparative research was most valid and reliable while clinical judgement and mechanical reasoning were less so. Such hierarchies are of limited value in health care. This is so because different assemblies of evidence are required to be considered in separate areas of health care; the evidence needed to make decisions related to public health differs from that required for clinical management of individual patients and therefore all of it cannot be accommodated in a single hierarchy. Neither is it valid in assessing evidence concerned with the care of individual patients because in relegating clinical judgement and mechanical reasoning it fails to acknowledge the fundamental importance of evidence derived from patients through clinical expertise on which all clinical decisions depend. The concept of a hierarchy of evidence applied to clinical care should be replaced by a system which acknowledges the primary importance of evidence obtained from individual patients.

In medicine, uncertainty is the norm and clinical decisions must be aimed at reducing it. The concept of evidence as a kind of truth cannot be justified. In reality, evidence is always open to interpretation and is frequently disputed due to differences in experience, knowledge and possible bias. Claims to unjustified authority based on singular interpretations of selections of evidence inevitably lead to conflicts.

Clinical guidelines have an important role in medicine. They require clinical expertise and judgement to be implemented in a manner which reflects the best interest of patients. Guidelines can only be advisory not commands. Clinicians must be aware of them and be prepared to follow them. However, implementing guidelines without reference to individual patient's needs and wishes is not appropriate and would not be an acceptable defence against harms caused by their use. Mechanical rules (predetermined rules made without reference to individual patients clinical circumstances) have no place in medicine.

Mechanistic reasoning based on understanding cause – effect relationships has an important role in medicine for example, in applying guidelines and clinical trial results to individual patients and in making clinical decisions where no guidelines and only limited evidence are available. Such reasoning is crucial evidence for developing scientific and ethical justification for the recruitment of patients to clinical trials. Inevitably, the use of mechanistic reasoning in clinical judgements features to a greater extent during the development of new treatments before high quality clinical trials have been conducted, declining in importance thereafter. Reliance on mechanistic reasoning as a sole basis for clinical decisions when good research evidence is available would be contrary to medical professionalism and regulatory requirements.

References

1. Howick J (2011). *The Philosophy of Evidence-Based Medicine*. Oxford: Wiley Blackwell BMJ Books.

2. Letter to GPs from Public Health England on The Use of Antivirals for the Treatment and Prophylaxis of Influenza. Available at: https://www.gov.uk/government/uploads/system/uploads/attachment_data/file/370676/Letter_to_clinicians.pdf (Accessed on 7/12/2015).

3. Cohen D (2015). GPs are Told to Treat with Septicism Advice on Anti-flu Drugs from Public Health England: *BMJ*, 350, h258.

4. Letter to GPs in the Thames Valley Area Re: Tamiflu for Prophylaxix of Influenza in Nursing and Care Homes. Available at: http://margaretmccartney.com/wp-content/uploads/2015/01/Tamiflu-letter.pdf Available from the author on request (Accessed on 7/12/2015).

5. Stiff GH. Re: GPs are Told to Treat with Scepticism Advice on Anti-flu Drugs from Public Health England. Available at: www.bmj.com/content/350/bmj.h258/rapid-responses (Accessed on 7/12/2015).

6. Cohen D (2015). BMA tells GPs to follow own Judgement in Prescribing Antiflu Drugs after Heated Row. *BMJ*, 350, h365.

7. Phin N. Re: GPs are Told to Treat with Scepticism Advice on Anti-flu Drugs from Public Health England. Available at: http://www.bmj.com/content/350/bmj.h258/rapid-responses (Accessed on 7/12/2015).

8. Carl HC, Jefferson T, Onakpoya I. Re: GPs are Told to Treat with Scepticism Advice on Anti-flu Drugs from Public Health England. Available at: http://www.bmj.com/content/350/bmj.h258/rapid-responses (Accessed on 7/12/2015).

9. Fryer C. Doctors can Depart from Guidelines in Patients' Best Interests. Available at: http://www.bmj.com/content/350/bmj.h417/rr; http://www.bmj.com/content/350/bmj.h841 (Accessed on 7/12/2015).

10. National Institute for Health Care and Excellence. Oseltamivir, Amantadine (Review) and Zanamivir for the Prophylaxis of Influenza. Available at:https://www.nice.org.uk/guidance/ta158 (Accessed on 7/12/2015).

11. Hoton R (2014). Offline: Statins — Where is the Leadership. *Lancet*, 384, 1561.

12. Measuring the Performance of The Cochrane Library. The Cochrane Library Oversight Committee. Available at: http://www.cochranelibrary.com/editorial/10.1002/14651858.ED000048 (Accessed on 7/12/2015).

13. Van Noorden R (2014). Report Disputes Benefit of Stock Piling Tamiflu. *Nature*. Available at: http://www.nature.com/news/report-disputes-benefit-of-stockpiling-tamiflu-1.15022 (Accessed on 7/12/2015).

14. McCartney M. Don't be bullied into prescribing Tamiflu. Available at: http://www.bmj.com/content/350/bmj.h417

15. Guyatt, GH (1991). Evidence-Based Medicine (Ed). American College of Physicians Journal Club. *Ann Int Med*, 114 (Suppl. 2), A16.

16. Evidence-Based Medicine Working Group (1992). Evidence-Based Medicine: A New Approach to Teaching the Practice of Medicine. *J Am Med Assoc*, 268, 2420–2425.

17. Oliver MF, Julian DG, Donald KW (1967). Problems in Evaluating Coronary Care Units. Their Responsibilities and their Relation to the Community. *Am J Cardiol*, 20, 465–474.

18. Julian DG (2001). The Evolution of the Coronary Care Unit. *Cardiovasc Res*, 51, 621–624.

19. Mather HG, Pearson NG, Read KLQ, Shaw DB, Steed GR, Thorne MG, Jones S, Guerrier CJ, Eraut CD, Mchugh PM, Chowdhury NR, Jafary MH, Wallace TJ (1971). Acute Myocardial Infarction: Home and Hospital Treatment. *BMJ*, 3, 334–338.

20. Mather HG, Morgan DC, Pearson NG, Thorne MG, Lawrence CJ, Riley IS (1976). Myocardial Infarction: A Comparison between Home and Hospital Care for Patients. *BMJ*, 1, 925–926.

21. Horrocks JC, Mccann AP, Staniland JR, Leaper DJ, De Dombal FT (1972). Computer-aided Diagnosis: Description of an Adaptable System, and Operational Experience with 2,034 Cases. *B Med J*, 2, 5–9.

22. De Dombal FT, Leaper DJ, Staniland JR, McCann AP, Horrocks JC (1972). Computer-Aided Diagnosis of Acute Abdominal Pain *B Med J*, 2, 9–13.

23. Available at: http://www.telegraph.co.uk/news/uknews/scotland/11317882/ Ebola-nurse-should-not-have-left-Heathrow-suggests-chief-medical-officer. html (Accessed on 7/12/2015).

24. Welsby PD (2014). Re: Ebola Virus Disease. *BMJ*, 349, g7348.

25. Sheridan DJ (2012). *Changes in Medical Professionalism in the 21st Century and Their Impact on Medical Science. In* Medical Science in the 21st Century Sunset Or New Dawn? London: Imperial College Press.

26. Stiell IG, McKnight RD, Greenberg GH, McDowell I, Nair RC, Wells GA, Johns C, Worthington JR (1994). Implementation of the Ottawa Ankle Rules. *JAMA*, 271, 827–832.

27. Stiell I, Wells G, Laupacis A, Brison R, Verbeek R, Vandemheen K, Naylor CD (1995). Multicentre Trial to Introduce the Ottawa Ankle Rules for Use of Radiography in Acute Ankle Injuries. Multicentre Ankle Rule Study Group. *BMJ*, 311 (7005), 594–597.

28. Jones TD, Bland EF (1935). Clinical Significance of Chorea as a Manifestation of Rheumatic Fever. A Study in Prognosis. *JAMA*, 451, 837.

29. Jones TD (1944). The Diagnosis of Rheumatic Fever. *JAMA*, 126(8), 481–484.

30. Antman EM, Lau J, Kupelnick B, Mosteller F, Chalmers TC (1992). A Comparison of Results of Meta-Analyses of Randomized Control Trials and Recommenda-

tions of Clinical Experts: Treatments For Myocardial Infarction. *JAMA*, 268(2), 240–248.

31. Rennie D, Chalmers I (2009). Assessing Authority. *JAMA*, 301, 1819–1821.

32. Haynes RB, Devereaux PJ, Guyatt GH (2002). Physicians' and Patients' Choices in Evidence Based Practice; Evidence does not make Decisions, People Do. *BMJ*, 324, 1350.

33. Chalmers I (2006). Why Fair Tests are Needed: A Brief History. *Evid Based Med*, 11, 67–68.

34. Preliminary Report (1989). Effect of Encainide and Flecainide on Mortality in a Randomized Trial of Arrhythmia Suppression after Myocardial Infarction. The Cardiac Arrhythmia Suppression Trial (CAST) Investigators. *N Engl J Med.*, 10: 321(6), 406–412.

35. Chalmers I (2007). Why Fair Tests are Needed: A Brief History. *Evid Based Nurs*, 10, 4–5.

36. Guyatt GH, Oxman AD, Vist GE, Kunz R, Falck-Ytter Y, Alonso-Coello P, Schünemann HJ (2008). An Emerging Consensus on Rating Quality of Evidence and Strength of Recommendations. *BMJ*, 336, 924–926.

37. Chalmers I (2006). Why Fair Tests are Needed: A Brief History. *ACP J Club.* 145(1), A8–A9.

38. Moore TJ (1995). *Deadly Medicine.* New York: Simon and Schuster.

39. Anderson JL, Pratt CM, Waldo AL, Karagounis LA (1997). Impact of the Food and Drug Administration Approval of Flecainide and Encainide on Coronary Artery Disease Mortality: Putting Deadly Medicine to the Test. *Am J Cardiol*, 79, 43–47.

40. Ferreira SH, Moncada S, Vane JR (1971). Indomethicin and Aspirin Abolish Prostaglandin Release from the Spleen. *Nat. New Biol*, 231, 237–239.

41. ISIS-2 (Second International Study of Infarct Survival) Collaboration Group. (1988). Randomised Trial of Intravenous Streptokinase, Oral Aspirin, both or neither among Cases of Suspected Acute Myocardial Infarction. *The Lancet*, 1, 397–402.

42. Velebit V, Podrid P, Lown B, Cohen BH, Graboys TB (1982). Aggravation and Provocation of Ventricular Arrhythmias by Antiarrhythmic Drugs. *Circulation*, 65, 886–892.

43. Winkle RA, Mason JW, Griffin JC (1982). Malignant Ventricular Tachyarrhythmias Associated with the Use of Encainide. *Am Heart J*, 102, 857–864.

44. Andersen H (2012). Mechanisms: What are they Evidence for in Evidence-based Medicine? *J Eval Clin Pract*, 18, 992–999.

45. Cohen AM, Stavri PZ, HirshWR (2003). A Categorization and Analysis of the Criticisms of Evidence-Based Medicine. *Int J Med Inform*, 73(1), 35–43.

Chapter 6

Evidenced-Based Medicine and Medical Science

Science explores what is unknown to discover new knowledge; Comparative research seeks the best of what is already known.

Evidence-Based Medicine (EBM) has become a major feature on the landscape of healthcare and has brought important advantages to medical practice. It also has the potential to impact widely on the environment in which medicine is practiced. This has significant implications for medical science which is intimately related to and dependent on that environment. In this chapter, I will explore the relationships between EBM and medical science and why the current model of EBM, which is largely based on epidemiological thinking and methods may be too narrow and a hindrance to medical science. I will use examples of past discoveries to illustrate how medical practice contributes to scientific advances; I will also use an example of a major challenge facing medicine today to illustrate how the impact of EBM may have changed the way this is being met.

Medical Science and Clinical Practice are Intimately Related and Interdependent

Medical science applies scientific methods to advance understanding of diseases and to find new cures for them. It is no longer possible to describe medical science easily in terms of the areas of investigation with which it is concerned. This is so because discoveries in many branches of science, which initially appear to have no relevance for medicine, can unexpectedly initiate new advances in diagnosis or treatment. For example piezoelectricity, the property whereby certain crystals change shape when a voltage is applied to them, was discovered in 1880 by Pierre and Jacque Curie and became the basis for developing ultrasound imaging in medicine. Wilhelm Roentgen's discoveries in 1895 similarly laid the foundations for X-ray diagnostic methods. Indeed, the number and range of advances in medicine that have resulted from discoveries in non-medical branches of science are so numerous that medical science is best thought of as a continuum of all the sciences. Convergence of the sciences is the inevitable result of expanding knowledge of the individual elements of it. This is implicitly recognised in new terminology such as "life sciences", which encompasses the study of all living organisms including microorganisms, plants, animals as well as humans. This is not just a bureaucratic reorganisation of academic research departments, but rather a reflection of how advances in knowledge have revealed shared evolutionary origins and molecular mechanisms among species. It also implies the hope that a wider collaboration among scientists will facilitate a more rapid application of new knowledge. So perhaps, a better description of medical science today would be the application of science without boundaries to improve understanding and treatment of human diseases, thus recognising human biology as part of nature and that knowledge of any part of it may have potential benefits.

This concept of science and knowledge without boundaries is not new. Indeed universities began as seats of learning to educate students in broad areas of science, philosophy and theology so that they became polymaths. This also implicitly recognised that solving specific problems was best achieved by drawing on broad areas of knowledge. However, as knowledge in science expanded after the Renaissance, it became increasingly difficult for students to become proficient in all areas and as a result specialisation was introduced. This facilitated greater expertise in limited areas and focused scientific research. It also contributed to more rapid expansion of knowledge and scientific discovery during the 19th Century. The discoveries of piezoelectricity and X-rays cited above are stunning examples of the benefits of such specialist scientific learning and research. However, finding ways to apply them to medicine required a less specialised system and perhaps something of a polymath approach. The development of ultrasound for imaging the heart illustrates this well. Although the Curie brothers discovered piezo-electricity in 1880,[1] it was not until 1953 when two Swedish scientists decided to investigate its possibilities for clinical uses. Inge Edler, a cardiologist based in Lund was looking for better ways to investigate diseases of the heart valves and Carl Hellmuth Hertz, a physicist at the University of Lund was familiar with the use of ultrasound for investigating fractures in materials. Edler initially conceived that a form of radar might be applicable. Discussions with Hertz who was familiar with ultrasound as a non-destructive method for detecting flaws in material led them to hypothesise that it might be used in humans.[2] They were able to test it using an ultrasound reflectoscope borrowed from a shipyard over a weekend in 1953, and showed that it could detect movement of the heart.[3] Based on this initial experience, they arranged for a long term loan of a machine to carry out a more detailed assessment, which showed beyond doubt its potential to image and diagnose cardiac valvular abnormalities. The emergence of new areas of research such as bioengineering and tissue engineering are a response to this. Medical science has of course many areas of interest including clinical science, pathology, psychiatry, pathology, molecular medicine to name a few. Clinical science refers to the search for new knowledge related to clinical practice. It is clinical in the sense that it investigates questions which arise from clinical practice; however, its methods are as likely to be based in the laboratory, for example, in molecular science, genetics and cell biology, as on the direct study of patients.

EBM: Impact on Science

EBM is related to but separate from medical science. EBM is not a science, but rather a concept that medical practice should be based on the best available evidence. It is related to science because much of that evidence is derived from science. It evolved as a process for distilling and comparing medical research, to determine what evidence best meets a particular need and is known as comparative research. A new branch of health research was developed in recent decades to undertake this task. The Cochrane Collaboration is the most widely known group who specialise in it and many of its founding members originated in the EBM movement. Medical science then could be said to explore the unknown to discover new knowledge; comparative research provides reviews of what is already known to determine what might best meet the needs of clinical practice. It is not a science therefore, but rather a filtering mechanism aimed at discerning which discoveries of science may be used to optimise the care of patients. In practice its remit has largely been concerned with evaluating new and existing treatments and hence, its impact is largely on clinical practice.

EBM has particular relevance for medical science for several reasons. Medical science and clinical practice are inextricably linked because the questions which the former seeks to address often arise from experience in clinical practice as does the motivation to find solutions for them. This is not to argue that clinicians should be the arbiters of what research is and is not done, or that they should be the priority setters for deciding what should be done. In recent years much discussion has centred on the need to involve a wide range of interested parties and stake holders in deciding research priorities, including governments, research funders, industry, journal editors and representatives of patient groups. Some might argue that setting priority areas for health including medical science is best achieved by consulting stakeholders[4,5] or by undertaking systematic reviews of literature to identify areas of need.[6] Others have argued that the traditional role of clinicians has been excessive and that their potential empire building aspirations amount to conflict of interest which should limit their role in setting priorities. This is part of the wider debate about how medical research should be funded and regulated, as discussed in Chapter 4. For medical science and clinical science in particular it has meant greater administrative control at the expense of science driven research. Irrespective of who decides medical research priorities, the diagnostic and therapeutic challenges that clinicians encounter inevitably provide a crucial impetus for asking the novel questions on which medical science depends. There are numerous examples of this in medicine[7] such as the development of ultrasound for clinical uses described above. It was the inadequacy of existing methods which Edler identified as a result of his clinical experience that led him to seek new and better techniques. The ability to question existing practice and to explore new methods in the context of clinical practice are crucial for medical science. It is for this reason that the way medicine is practiced and its intellectual environment are so important for medical science. This in turn is why the rhetoric of the EBM movement and its potential impact on clinical practice are relevant and important to clinical science.

Progress in clinical science, as indeed all science depends on knowledge of the area under investigation, hypothesis making, collecting evidence and reasoning. Just as these are essential for clinical practice, as discussed in Chapter 5, they are also fundamental to all original scientific work. The development of medical ultrasound discussed above illustrates this. It was clinical experience of inadequate diagnostic methods that sparked Edler's initial curiosity and his collaboration with Hertz knowledge as a physicist which led them to hypothesise that it might be used in humans. This example shows the importance of the intellectual environment in which clinical practice is based, the ability to ask questions, space for curiosity to flourish and opportunities to explore hypotheses for medical science to flourish.

Medical Science: Data Sets versus Hypothesis and Reasoning

An alternative view is that such hands-on experience is now less important to advance medical science and that accumulation of large population data sets is more productive than hypothesis making and reasoning. This argument is used to justify large data gathering operations with the intention of creating banks of data which can subsequently be "mined" to test unspecified hypotheses in the future. In the life sciences this typically involves collecting lifestyle information together with blood samples for genetic analysis from large samples of representative populations. They require large investments and several countries have now set up their own national "Biobanks". They invariably attract criticism and debate[8-10] since their potential value cannot be easily assessed at the outset and even their design and management are problematic, since their potential for future use cannot be fully understood in advance. Their real value will only emerge with time. In contrast, there has long been very wide agreement among plant biologists on the value and importance of storing and preserving botanical specimens such as the millennium seed bank project.[11] The latter, however, is also highly motivated by the need for conservation amid concerns that many plant species are becoming extinct and opportunities to study them in the future may not be possible.

John Snow's Discovery of Water Borne Cholera: Truth is Richer than Myth

The idea that discoveries are made principally by interpreting data rather than hypothesis making and reasoning is supported by misleading reconstructions of how important discoveries have been made. This may result from attempts to provide simplified descriptions by omitting much of the detailed work in order to make them more comprehensible. It can also be the result of straight forward mythmaking. A good example of the latter is the discovery by John Snow in 1850s that cholera is spread by drinking contaminated water. Snow was a physician and a founder of anaesthesia who took a deep interest in cholera epidemics. He was remarkable for his conclusion that cholera was spread by drinking contaminated water because it was at odds with the prevailing view at the time and was contradicted by a major officially funded research. He is widely believed to have made his discovery as a result of his drawing a map of deaths related to a particular water pump during an epidemic in the Golden Square area of London. This is often hailed as an example of the power of data collection and the founding action of the science of epidemiology.[12] But it is in fact a myth which obscures the actual methods he used. It is helpful therefore to consider how he studied the problem and how he reached his conclusion. A careful study of his work[13] showed clearly that Snow had already developed and tested his hypothesis that cholera was a water borne disease long before he drew his map. He had reasoned that cholera was an illness of the gut and that its symptoms were due to fluid loss and that infection was by mouth and spread was by the faecal-oral route.[14] Before the outbreak of cholera in the Golden Square area he had learned that water provided to a large area of south London was supplied by two competing companies, one of which drew its source from a polluted section of the Thames whereas the other moved its intake to a higher and cleaner area. He decided to use this information to test his hypothesis that contaminated water was causing the spread of cholera by studying mortality rates due to cholera in relation to the supply of water. He had been engaged in that work when the Golden Square outbreak occurred and decided to interrupt it for a short period to investigate the water supplied by the five pumps in Golden Square. By relating deaths to pump locations he was able to identify the Broad Street pump as the most likely source of contaminated water.[14] In order to illustrate his conclusion, Snow produced a map of deaths in the area around Golden Square in London in 1854 showing their close proximity in relation to the Broad Street water pump. This was in contrast to much fewer deaths among residents living close to other pumps in the area. Snow later informed the Board of Guardians of St. James Parish who arranged for the handle of the pump to be removed.[15] His map was undoubtedly important in helping to convince local officials about the need to disable the pump. But it was not the basis of his conclusion that cholera was a water-borne disease.

It is clear then that Snow had already deduced that contaminated water was the most likely source of the cholera infection from his earlier work prior to the Golden Square outbreak and not from the map he had prepared.[16] It was his conclusions based on this earlier work that led him directly to investigate water supplies in the Golden Square outbreak. His decision to illustrate his findings in a map followed from and was a consequence of this. Snow's map was intended to confirm what he had already deduced; it was not the primary reason for his conclusions. The importance of his earlier work is also supported by the fact that maps of deaths due to cholera in relation to water supplies and sewage works had been produced by others who drew different conclusions to those of Snow.[14] Snow's map contained no information which he had not already tabulated; however, its visual impact would have been considerable and would have been useful in explaining his conclusion to local officials. This is reminiscent of Florence Nightingale's use of diagrams and statistical data to convey her message so as to "effect thro the eyes what we may fail to convey to the brains of the public through their word proof ears". He first published his map at a meeting of the Epidemiological Society in London in 1854,[14] and included it in the second edition of his book.[16] Thus, Snow's map was a powerful visual confirmation of what he had already deduced. It was also useful as a means of communication and advocating his conclusion, but it was not the basis on which he reached it.

An interesting discussion of how Snow arrived at his conclusions about cholera suggests that he not only based them on reasoning methods, but that he was aware of the importance of using accepted formal reasoning principles.[17] For example, in reasoning that cholera was transmissible from person to person, Snow noted the following cases; "Mrs. N. went from Paul, a village close to the Humber, to Hedon, two miles off, to nurse her brother in cholera;

the next day, after his death, went to nurse Mrs. B., also at Hedon; within two days was attacked herself; was removed to a lodging house; the son of the lodging-house keeper was attacked the next day, and died. Mrs. N.'s son removed her back to Paul; was himself attacked two days afterwards, and died." He then went on to comment as follows, "It would be easy, by going through the medical journals and works which have been published on cholera, to quote as many cases similar to the above as would fill a large volume. But the above instances are quite sufficient to show that cholera can be communicated from the sick to the healthy; for it is quite impossible that even a 10th part of these cases of consecutive illness could have followed each other by mere coincidence, without being connected as cause and effect"[16] (p. 9). He thus invokes what philosophers call the no-miracle argument to draw his conclusion, meaning, it would be too much of a coincidence (or a miracle) if these cases were not linked by cause and effect. A further example of Snow's awareness of reasoning principles was in his avoidance of ad hoc modifications of his hypothesis. If a theory is likely to be true then it should not be necessary to make changes to it in order to explain unexpected observations. One example of this is the seasonal variation in cholera which Snow had observed and sought to explain, "Each time when cholera has been introduced into England in the autumn, it has made but little progress, and has lingered rather than flourished during the winter and spring, to increase gradually during the following summer, reach its climax at the latter part of summer, and decline somewhat rapidly as the cool days of autumn set in. In most parts of Scotland, on the contrary, cholera has each time run through its course in the winter immediately following its introduction"[16] (p. 117). Snow saw this as unexpected behaviour which he was obliged to reconcile with his theory of water borne transmission. Rather than modify his hypothesis he instead put forward the following explanation. "The English people, as a general rule, do not drink much unboiled water, except in warm weather. They generally take tea, coffee, malt liquor, or some other artificial beverage at their meals, and do not require to drink between meals, except when the weather is warm. In summer, however, a much greater quantity of drink is required, and it is much more usual to drink water at that season than in cold weather." He explained the differences between England and Scotland as follows, "In Scotland, on the other hand, unboiled water is somewhat freely used at all times to mix with spirits; I am told that when two or three people enter a tavern in Scotland and ask for a gill of whiskey, a jug of water and tumbler-glasses are brought with it. Malt liquors are only consumed to a limited extent in Scotland, and when persons drink spirit without water, as they often do, it occasions thirst and obliges them to drink water afterwards"[16] (p. 118). Snow was aware that, the fact that he could explain this behaviour without modifying his hypothesis increased its likelihood of being true.

A further example of Snow's use of formal reasoning principles is in what is known as the method of difference. The concept here is that when two contradictory observations have everything in common except one aspect, then the cause is likely to be related to that single difference. Snow used this argument to show that cholera was caused by polluted water in cases of cholera which occurred in 1849 in Thomas Street, Horsleydown. Here there were two adjacent courts, in which the houses occupying the north side of one and the south side of the other were placed back to back, separated by a small area in which the privies of each were located. Although there were 11 deaths in 7 of the 14 houses on the south side of this drain, there was only one case in the adjoining houses to the north of it. Investigating these cases, Snow observed that; "In the former court, the slops of dirty water, poured down by the inhabitants into a channel in front of the houses, got into the well from which they obtained their water; this being the only difference that Mr. Grant, the Assistant-Surveyor for the Commissioners of Sewers, could find between the circumstances of the two courts, as he stated in a report that he made to the Commissioners"[16] (p. 23). Here Snow identifies the *only difference* between the houses to explain the higher mortality, invoking Mill's principle of differences.[17] His work illustrates the power of reasoning in deducing the cause of cholera when there was no way to confirm it. It is also noteworthy that his conclusions were in fact at odds with the most widely held theory that cholera was caused by miasmas and spread by effluvia.

This case is important because it demonstrates the weakness of relying exclusively on data to draw conclusions. For Snow generating the data on which he made his map was secondary to and necessitated the application of careful reasoning. If he had waited for data without applying reason it may never have appeared. Understanding the ways in which discoveries are made is also important for medicine and particularly so in discussing EBM, because of the role attributed to data analysis by the EBM movement and its criticism of mechanistic reasoning. In its efforts to promote better practice, the EBM movement emphasised the importance of trial data above reasoning in its hierarchy of evidence as discussed in Chapter 5. If this were taken at face value it would tend to move clinical practice towards a data driven technical exercise by relegating the clinical evidence obtained from patients, and would undermine the human aspect of care. To some, this might appear a more efficient use of medical manpower in hard pressed health care systems facing high levels of demand. In such circumstances, it might even be considered beneficial to focus on increasing productivity and efficiency by controlling anything which appears to impair meeting immediate delivery targets, for example by controlling research leading to new and potentially costly innovations,[18] or by advocating a simplified data driven care system based on a restrictive hierarchy of evidence. However, it would risk undermining medical science and is contrary to the professional responsibilities of physicians which include preserving knowledge and discovering new knowledge through engagement in science. It is noteworthy that at the time Snow made his enquiries a large officially directed and funded research program was undertaken into the problem by the Board of Health. This amassed a large amount of data related to air temperature and pressure, wind direction, cloud cover, fog, rainfall, Thames water temperature as well as details of cholera deaths and their locations. However, unlike Snow's method it lacked any clear hypothesis or strategy to test one. It rejected Snow's conclusions in favour of the more popular miasmatic theory for the spread of cholera.[19] Snow's methods then demonstrate the power of principled reasoning based on a thorough grounding in pathophysiology applied to a major medical challenge; indeed, data without reason becomes a fog. They also show the value of maintaining clinical practice in an environment which encourages a sense of enquiry based on knowledge, experience and training in the methods of original science. Snow's motivation appears to have been largely intrinsic and borne out of his knowledge, intelligence and sense of enquiry. Progress in medical science will depend on harnessing this in our own time.

Snow is often described as the founder of the methods of epidemiology. This principally relates to his presentation of the data he collected and his use of statistical methods. The original launch of the EBM movement was also based largely on epidemiology, in which most of its founders were experts. It stressed the importance of epidemiological methods of data collection and statistical analysis and advocated these as superior evidence compared to clinical observation and pathophysiological reasoning. However, as discussed above, Snow's contribution to medical science went far beyond such methods. As we have seen, his success depended on the use of mechanistic reasoning grounded in pathophysiology. He was also a physician and a pioneer of anaesthesia.[20,21] Furthermore, all of Snow's work can be seen as a drive to improve health, either by understanding better the nature and causes of illness, or by improving methods to treat it. He identified gaps on the state of knowledge of disease and treatments available in his time and sought to improve them for the future. In this respect, his outlook differs markedly from the current epidemiological approach to EBM; the latter is much more focused on making the best use of what is available now, rather than exploring new horizons. It uses the methods of comparative research to evaluate and prioritise current knowledge. Snow's work was closer to that of original science, exploring the unknown to discover new knowledge. This distinction also underlies some potentially negative effects on medical science of the current epidemiological model of EBM.

Data without Reason becomes a Fog

Treating patients today must be based on the best of what is currently available. No doubt, many new treatments will emerge in the future but they cannot be foreseen. It makes sense therefore that, EBM is based on what is known. However, a healthcare environment which is overly or exclusively focused on evaluating the current state of knowledge may have difficulty in foreseeing and meeting future challenges. As discussed in Chapter 3, the task of evaluating and maintaining up to date reviews of the large body of medical research published each year is formidable and a major commitment. It is also a task which has become even more important for hard pressed healthcare delivery systems facing economic challenges and seeking greater efficiency and cost effectiveness. However, if our efforts to meet today's needs become all-consuming we will fail to foresee future challenges and grasp opportunities to meet them, and there are signs that this may already be happening.

The Problem of Antibiotic Resistance

Alexander Fleming, Ernst Chain and Howard Florey received jointly the Nobel Prize in 1945 for their discovery of penicillin. In their Nobel lectures at the time, both Fleming and Florey drew attention to the reality of antibiotic resistance. Fleming noted the dangers of exposing bacteria to doses of penicillin insufficient to kill them, but which allowed them to develop resistance and emphasised that "if you use penicillin, use enough".[22] Florey also was aware that streptomycin was capable of inducing high resistance in susceptible organisms and that "its clinical use will not be quite so straight forward as one could hope".[23] Their warnings seem largely to have gone unheard, and medicine entered a "golden era" of antibiotic use from the 1930s to 1960s with a seemingly endless supply of new drug resistant antibiotics. However, during the past two decades antibiotic resistance has emerged as one of the great global health challenges of our time. In January 2015, President Obama announced his commitment to increase funding to $1.2 billion from 2016 to combat the problem.[24] In 2014, the UK Government commissioned economist Jim O'Neill to enquire into the problem. His review published in December 2014 and backed by reports prepared by two consultant agencies highlighted potential catastrophic consequences of the problem, estimating that 300 million people might die as a result of antibiotic resistant infections during the next 35 years with a 2–3.5% reduction in global GDP.[25] The European Union is also engaged with the problem of funding new research and efforts to conserve the effectiveness of existing drugs.[26] The problem of antibiotic resistance is perpetual; it is built into the genetic make-up of bacteria, their mutation and high replication rates making them ideally suited to develop resistance. Joshua Lederberg who won the Nobel Prize for his work on bacterial genetics described the challenge as "our wits versus their genes",[27] just as Florey saw that the development of resistance to streptomycin would complicate and limit its use 55 years earlier. It makes sense therefore that solutions to it need to address several areas, in particular conserving the effectiveness of current stocks of antibiotics, and in developing new ones to replace those no longer effective.

Contrasting US and UK Approaches

Healthcare services in most western countries face challenges of increasing demand and rising costs and consequently medical science must compete for limited resources among other pressing demands. Challenges such as antibiotic resistance are global in nature and how we respond to them reflects the conditions which prevail in each country. In the US, the president's response to the problem was based on a report[28] by his council of advisors on science and technology, a group of the nation's leading scientists and engineers. The plan would double funding to combat the problem to around $1,200 million of which 54% would go to develop new antibiotics and rapid diagnostic tests, 23% would promote responsible use of antibiotics so as to conserve their effectiveness, 13% would be used to reduce resistance in health care settings and 4% would be given to the Federal Drug Administration to support the evaluation of new antibiotic and to phase out their use in food production.[24] In the UK, the response to the problem was quite different. The predominant concern is with the over-use and inappropriate use of the present stock of antibiotics and the need to conserve them; priority is given to preventing infections, increased surveillance of infections and antibiotic use, education and training.[29] Challenges to the development of new antibiotics are seen predominantly as logistic, economic and uncertainty about the regulatory environment for drug approval; in essence, problems faced by the pharmaceutical industry. On-going research in academia is noted and the need to prioritise future work is advocated, but with little new investment.[29] All of these are laudable and important steps and there is no doubt that antibiotics are over pre-scribed.[30] They are also emblematic of the predominant approach to health-care challenges in the UK based on the current model of EBM — making the best of what we have now. But they also show a glaring gap in our willingness to engage seriously with medical science to find future solutions. It seems as if our policy makers have become so blinded by the rhetoric and promise of EBM and the obviousness of making the best of what we have now, that the possibilities of what science might bring for the future are no longer visible. It is also striking in this context that in contrast to the scientific approach in the US, the main UK Government enquiry into the problem was headed by an economist backed by two consulting agencies. There seems to have been little involvement of scientists and none of the reports it produced were subject to external peer review.[25] And yet, the only secure long term approach will have to be based on the fact that all current antibiotics will eventually become unusable, given the proficiency of bacterial genetics. Therefore, the need to find new and better ways to diagnose and treat bacterial infections is inescapable, and this ultimately will depend on advances in science.

How Penicillin was Discovered and Developed

It is relevant here to recall how penicillin was discovered and made available for clinical use. Fleming was working as a bacteriologist with the ability to undertake research alongside his service. He was well aware as indeed it was generally known at the time that microbial antagonisms were commonplace, as he explained "it is seldom that an observant clinical bacteriologist can pass a week without seeing in the course of his ordinary work very definite instances of bacterial antagonism".[22] Fleming had studied the bacteriology of many cases of gas gangrene during the WWI,[31] and was aware of the limitations of antiseptic treatment of wounds. His first hand experience of such infections would have left him in no doubt about the potential benefit of effective antimicrobial treatments and this would have motivated his later work in this area as a bacteriologist. And so, he noticed the powerful bactericidal properties of lysozyme in 1921.[32] His discovery of penicillin was based on a chance observation when a culture plate growing colonies of *staphylococci* became contaminated by a mould. He noticed that the *staphylococci* colonies around the mould colony were being destroyed and he knew that it was important observation. He decided to investigate it further by isolating and examining the mould, which turned out to be a member of the genus penecillium. He was able to grow the mould in a pure form and confirmed its bactericidal properties against several different bacteria. He then grew the mould in a liquid culture and showed that the antibacterial effect was present in the culture medium. He compared the effect with that of lysozyme and noticed that although the effects were similar they acted against different strains of bacteria; whereas lysozyme destroyed many bacteria that are harmless to humans, penicillin killed several important human pathogens.[22,33]

Full development of penicillin as a clinically useful antibiotic required the production of larger quantities which Fleming was unable to achieve. Ernst Chain, Howard Florey and colleagues working in Oxford some years later succeeded in preparing a sufficient amount to treat a single seriously ill patient with a positive response. Although the patient subsequently relapsed and died as their supply ran out, they were convinced of its potential clinical use. Their publication in 1940 demonstrating a convincing therapeutic response[34] galvanised research. Chain and his colleagues went on to characterise the chemical structure of penicillin[35] and later Dorothy Hodgkin also working at Oxford using X-ray crystallography confirmed the structure they surmised. Although Florey and Chain greatly increased the production of penicillin, their yields were still far too low for general clinical use. A UK and US government agreement to share information in order to facilitate scaling up production led to the introduction of commercial industrial methods based on deep fermentation processes available in the US. This greatly increased yields and by 1945, over 600 billion units per year were being produced. Penicillin is a good example of how successful advances in medicine emerge and are successfully exploited. There is no doubt that, WWII was a powerful impetus for the rapid expansion of work on penicillin after 1939 and in particular the rapid and successful adoption of methods for mass production. However, none of this would have been possible without the earlier work which established the knowledge on which it was based. How did this come about and what were the circumstances in which it occurred?

Fleming went to some lengths to explain how he made his discovery.[22] He accounted for it as a chance observation and was particular in clarifying that it would be untrue if he had claimed that it was the result of "serious study of the literature and deep thought that, valuable antibacterial substances were made by moulds and that I set out to investigate the problem". He acknowledged that, his "only merit is that I did not neglect the observation and that I pursued the subject as a bacteriologist". How was he able to make the observation and what prompted him to pursue it rather than neglect it as others had done? After all, as he tells us "To my generation of bacteriologists the inhibition of one microbe by another was commonplace. We were all taught about these inhibitions and indeed it is seldom that an observant clinical bacteriologist can pass a week without seeing in the course of his ordinary work very definite instances of bacterial antagonism". I suggest that the answers to these questions can be found in Fleming's earlier experience. He had first-hand experience of seriously infected wounds as a clinical bacteriologist during WWI. This had allowed him to investigate the bacteriology of wounds complicated by gas gangrene, a particularly serious infection caused by gas producing bacteria.[31] We can tell from his publication of this work that he was well trained in bacteriology and in research methods. He must also have been motivated by a sense of enquiry, no doubt reinforced by his clinical experience. He would certainly have been in no doubt about the importance of discovering how to combat organisms causing such infections. In this context, a key aspect of his chance observation was that the bacteria being destroyed by the contaminating mould were *staphylococci*, which he knew well to be a serious human pathogen. Fleming then was trained in medicine and as a scientist. He was alert to the importance of new knowledge in his field and committed to discovery. He could be said to fulfil the conditions in the quotation attributed to Louis Pasteur "In the fields of observation chance favours only the prepared mind". Looked at in this way, Flemings observation and his scientific pursuit of it make perfect sense.

Taking up the task in 1939, Chain, a trained chemist, was able to extract sufficient material to test penicillin in animals and to show that it was non-toxic. Florey who was head of the Sir William Dunn School of Pathology in Oxford saw its importance and the need to assemble a team with wide ranging skills to take it forward. He was able to do this because the Dunn School already had scientists with such skills and the facilities for laboratory work needed to scale-up production and test its efficacy in animals. He also arranged collaboration with physicians at the nearby Radcriffe Infirmary to undertake early trials in patients with serious infections. It was the dramatic success of these early tests which led to negotiations between the UK and US Governments, and the scaling up of mass production. As Florey expressed it, success depended "on the development and co-ordinated use of technical methods", and taking advantage of advances in biochemistry, which "has been acquiring new techniques, often of great delicacy, suitable for dealing with many substances which occur naturally".

Meeting the Challenge; Then and Now

These events which led to the discovery of penicillin and the circumstances which enabled them differ sharply from the conditions we find today almost a century later facing the challenge of discovering new antibiotics. Whereas the focus then was on scientific research exemplified by the work of Fleming, Chain and Florey, all of whom were highly motivated scientists who combined laboratory and clinical skills in a well-coordinated and effective manner. Scaling up the mass production of penicillin required industrial methods; this was understood immediately and agreements put in place to facilitate it. It is ironic that in the UK where these initial discoveries were made the conditions and prospects for new discoveries now seem far less promising. The emphasis is predominantly on conserving the antibiotics we have, and trying to identify and create economic conditions that might encourage the pharmaceutical industry to develop new drugs. An enquiry by UK members of parliament[36] emphasised the problem of inappropriate use and poor stewardship of antibiotics in health care and farming, and the need for decisive action to prevent this. The failure to discover new antibiotics was considered essentially as an issue of the pharmaceutical industry's poor pipeline and the solutions recommended were almost entirely concerned with adjusting the market conditions for pharmaceuticals to encourage the industry. The committee received written advice from 66 organisations and heard evidence from senior leaders of the department of health, medicine, industry, health care management and a wide range of related organisations. The source of its advice can truly be said to be democratic and representative of a wide range of stakeholders. However, evidence sought from leading scientists who are actively engaged in the search and aware of the scientific challenges and prospects for finding new antibiotics was minimal.[36] The committee agreed with the Government's strategy that introducing economic measures to encourage the pharmaceutical industrial was the key priority to ensuring the development of new antibiotics.[25] This is based on the fact that antibiotics are prescribed for relatively short periods and therefore are less profitable than drugs used to treat chronic conditions and this together with the high costs of development has been a deterrent to the industry.

These are sensible measures in the short term, however, the experience of developments such as penicillin suggest that they are unlikely to lead to the advances in knowledge needed to replace our present antibiotics. The pharmaceutical industry has been remarkably successful in scaling up and bringing to market many new antibiotics; however, these were largely variants of previous drugs. Its record in developing new antibiotics based on novel mechanisms to combat resistant microbes has been poor and this failure together with the high costs involved led them to pursue other targets. This is not a surprise and neither is it a criticism of the industry. It is simply a reflection of the fact that all businesses including pharmaceutical companies are motivated and driven by economic priorities. The manner in which penicillin production was so rapidly scaled-up is an excellent example of what they can achieve. However, this was based on developments in fermentation processes and had little to do with the science of antimicrobials. It took forward the scientific advances which had been made and showed how separately developed industrial processes could be used to bring it to market. The pharmaceutical industry undertakes a great deal of research; however, the vast majority of this is either routine screening procedures or work to meet regulatory requirements. Its contribution to expanding fundamental knowledge is far less.[37] It is difficult to envisage how the industry alone can be relied on to undertake the fundamental research needed to meet the long term challenge. This is also implicit in the US response where the evidence gathered and proposals put forward are predominantly geared to advancing scientific research. In contrast in the UK, most effort is centred on healthcare management strategies and economic adjustments.

It seems surprising given its past successes in medical science such as the discovery of penicillin that the UK has now chosen to leave medical science in the background. There may be several reasons for this. There has been a long term acknowledgement and concern that many past successes in science in the UK have failed to lead to economic successes at home and of course penicillin is another example of this. This tends to be misconstrued as a failure of science to take development from the laboratory forward and to a sense that the effort and investment has failed to reap expected benefits. But as we saw in the case of penicillin, its commercial development was based on utilising existing industrial fermentation technology in the US. Had such an opportunity been available in the UK, there is no reason to suppose it would have gone abroad. It is misconception to see this as a failure of science; rather it reflects our limited industrial capacity for investing in new technologies. Nevertheless, the view persists and may contribute to a negative attitude towards science. A second possible reason is the change in organisation and administration of medical science in the UK during the past three decades. As discussed in Chapter 4, administration and regulation of medical science is now centred more within the department of health in order to meet its priorities and research needs. This inevitably shifted the focus away from traditional science-led-science, of the kind Fleming and Florey were able to undertake and more towards the immediate healthcare delivery needs of the department; indeed, the recommendations of the

House of Commons Committee on Science and Technology fit those short term needs well. It has also tended to distance basic medical sciences from the clinical arena.

Problems Seeking Solutions versus Solutions Seeking Problems

Research in life sciences in the UK continues to be highly successful academically[38] and in attracting foreign investment.[39] Despite this there is increasing public concern that advances in biology are not helping patients adequately. Leaders of life sciences are concerned that developments in genomics, data analysis and e-technologies have the potential to transform health care but have not been embraced by medical innovation process and as a result opportunities such as personalised medicines are not being developed.[40] They identify a failure of coordinated action between service users, health professionals, service providers and innovators and the need for "transformative thinking" to ensure that they "pull together". It is surely an extraordinary irony of our times that in addressing the problem of antibiotic resistance, one of our most pressing challenges in healthcare, the potential contribution of science is marginalised. And yet we now have great technological advances in life sciences struggling to find opportunities in medicine. This of course was not a problem for Snow or Fleming because they were deeply involved in both science and clinical care. They in effect embodied the translation of discoveries in the laboratory to clinical care. That link is now much weakened by the growing separation of medicine and science, which I suggest is a major factor in the current translation gap. Physicians are no longer sufficiently involved in the dual processes of science and care. Doctors are concerned with diagnosing and treating sick patients and their interests and motivation will most often reflect this. Most will struggle to see the point of personalised medicines unless they are directed towards meeting a treatment or diagnostic challenge they encounter, such as new effective antibiotics. Calls for a new social contract to improve medical innovation[40] will only work if it includes a restoration of the role of the physician-scientist more widely, to help guide life sciences to tackle real therapeutic challenges and to identify advances in science which can be used to improve diagnosis and treatment.

The current epidemiological model of EBM may have contributed to the growing gap between medicine and science. The EBM movement's concept of a hierarchy of evidence-based predominantly on previously published research and its relegation of mechanistic reasoning, knowledge and experience are fundamentally contrary to the way original science works. Although these views have been discredited and are now largely abandoned by the movement they contributed to an atmosphere in which rules and guideline-following in medicine can appear more important than maintaining a sense of enquiry and the motivation to pursue unexplained observations. As discussed in Chapter 3, members of the EBM movement mounted a campaign, accusing the science community of waste on a vast scale. More recently, the idea of "evidence-based research" has been proposed[6] and a new campaign mounted to advocate the greater use of comparative research methods in primary research by pressing "funders, regulators, researchers, academic institutions and journals to ensure that scientists should learn the methodology of systematic reviews". On the face of it, this sounds plausible. However, activism of this kind can also be harmful. When the case being pressed is narrow and fails to acknowledge other important issues, it risks distorting how priorities are perceived and how science works. In this context, it is helpful to recall Fleming's comment about his discovery of penicillin, "I might have claimed that I had come to the conclusion, as a result of serious study of the literature and deep thought, that valuable antibacterial substances were made by moulds and that I set out to investigate the problem. That would have been untrue and I preferred to tell the truth that penicillin started as a chance observation". Original science is an exploratory process much dependent on the intrinsic motivation of individuals. Progress and the direction it follows are often unpredictable since these depend on what new knowledge emerges and chance observations have always been an important part of it. Systematic reviews are a valuable research tool and they have an important place in medicine. They can also be useful for scientists in reviewing past research. They are however, just one tool of many that are useful. The suggestion that they are a prerequisite for any and all scientific experiments is wrong and represents a distorted view about how original science works. While it would be foolish to design a clinical trial in a well-researched area without undertaking a careful review of what has been done previously, much original science is undertaken in areas where the established knowledge is contained in the minds of a handful of scientists and a formal systematic review even if possible would be a wasteful paper exercise. Activism has a place in medicine; however, the over-arching emphasis on systematic reviews in this new campaign embodies a similarly restricted view of evidence to that advocated by the EBM movement a quarter of a century ago and fails for the same reasons as discussed in Chapter 5. It also shifts the emphasis in science towards administration, regulation and oversight and away from the actual questions science seeks to address. Science becomes more about how it is done rather than what it actually does. This is well exemplified in current issues of widely read medical journals. Whereas a century ago they contained the discoveries of Fleming, Chain and Florey,[31,34] the priority today concerns the politics, administration and regulation of science with apparently little interest in the science itself.[40,41] This is symptomatic of a growing separation between clinical medicine and science which has emerged during the 21st century. It is also hindering medical progress by undermining the links which help to direct scientific effort towards clinical problems and to recognise the clinical potential of advances in science. And so, it is hardly surprising then that we find less engagement with science, loss of trust in what it can achieve and that we have scientists championing major advances but finding apparently little appetite to explore their potential utility in medicine. On the other hand, we face major challenges in diagnosis and treatment, of which antibiotic resistance is just one, and yet the possibilities which science can bring to meet them are marginalised. There are many reasons for this which I have discussed previously.[42] These include the seemingly endless stream of well-intentioned but failed healthcare reforms aimed at increasing efficiency and productivity, which have forced medical science from the clinical agenda and increasingly into isolated laboratories.

The present model of EBM I suggest, also contributed to this dilemma. With its heavy reliance on epidemiological thinking and methods, it has contributed, to an overwhelming focus on the present and past. Its efforts are singularly directed towards the analysis of what has gone before and its output supports an increasingly regulated clinical environment. While there are some benefits in this, it has also contributed to a box-ticking and overmanaged clinical work force, increasingly concerned that it is being driven by data instead of patients' needs. It also creates a false sense of security by promoting the concept that the answers to diagnostic and therapeutic questions can be found in analysing data from the past. When these are formulated into authoritative guidelines it tends to undermine the need to question what might be better and to seek more effective treatments. Some may see this as beneficial in producing a more efficient and less distracted workforce. However, as discussed in Chapter 5 it is also leading to disputes, and as I have suggested here it is harming medical science. EBM is a good thing, but it needs to be rooted more broadly in medicine and medical science. At present the EBM movement continues to be one principally of advocacy based on epidemiology, public health and statistics with too few of its advocates having hands-on experience in clinical care or original science, and its understanding of them may consequently be limited.

Conclusions

Medical science and clinical practice are intimately related and interdependent. Consequently, the way medicine is practiced and its environment are important. EBM was developed to improve clinical practice by providing reliable reviews of clinical trials and thereby more up-to-date evidence. Progress in medical science often depends on clinicians being willing and able to question treatments and diagnostic methods and to explore possible new approaches. These depend on hypothesis making and reasoning based on sound knowledge of biological mechanisms and experience. The present model of EBM is heavily weighted towards epidemiology and statistical methods applied to existing knowledge. Its founders favoured a hierarchy of evidence based on such data and questioned the reliability of reasoning and experience in clinical practice. While the value of clinical trial data is undisputed in medicine, an over reliance of such data at the expense of clinical evidence obtained from patients and reasoning is increasingly recognised as harmful to medicine and patients. It is also harmful for medical science. Numerous examples of past discoveries in medical science illustrate the importance of hypotheses and principled reasoning and that data without them can reveal little. It is vital therefore that these are preserved in medicine.

Healthcare delivery in most western countries faces increasing demand and rising costs. Efforts to increase efficiency and productivity have made it more difficult for physicians to be involved in science. The present epidemiological model of EBM may have contributed to this by promoting the concept of greater clinical efficiency based on a simplified data driven model of practice. This has caused an increasing separation of medical practice and science. Consequences of this are evident in the fact that advances in life sciences are struggling to find roles in medicine while at the same time administrative and economic solutions are prioritised in meeting major medical challenges, such as antibiotic resistance. This disengagement appears more prominent in the UK where EBM is also strongest. These are serious threats to the future of medicine and medical science. They have of course many causes, but the present model of EBM is one of them due to its failure to embrace medicine and medical science more widely and by its over-reliance on epidemiological thinking and methods. Too few of its founders and advocates have been sufficiently hands-on clinicians or engaged in original science.

The concept of EBM is an important contribution to medicine in refocusing attention on the need for careful evaluation of published evidence. It has much to contribute in the future. However, caring for patients requires more than is possible through the analysis of data. It also requires and obliges physicians to be mindful of and committed to the search for new ways to diagnose and treat patients. Progress in medical science is now facing the paradoxical challenge of being rich in technological advances, but lacking the skills to guide their development to fit clinical needs and to grasp the possibilities that currently exist. A concept of EBM more broadly based in clinical practice and original science, one that is not satisfied to rely on what is already known, but recognises the need for new knowledge and evidence would be one step on the road to reversing this.

References

1. Curie P, Curie J (1880). Developpement, Par Pression de l'electricite Polaire Dans les Cristaux Hemiedres A Faces Inclinees. *Comptes Rendus*, 91, 291–295.
2. Marsal K (2001). In Memoriam: Inge Edler — The Father of Echocardiography. *Eur J Ultrasound*, 13, 179–182.
3. Edler I, Lindström K (2004). The History of Echocardiography. *Ultrasound Med Biol*, 30(12),1565–1644.
4. Scuffham PA, Ratcliffe J, Kendall E, Burton P, Wilson A, Chalkidou K, Littlejohns P, Whitty JA (2014). Engaging the Public in Healthcare Decision-Making: Quantifying Preferences for Healthcare through Citizens' Juries. *BMJ Open*, 2; 4(5), doi: 10.1136/bmjopen-2014-005437.

5. Ioannidis JP, Greenland S, Hlatky MA, Khoury MJ, Macleod MR, Moher D, Schulz KF, Tibshirani R (2014). Increasing Value and Reducing Waste in Research Design, Conduct, and Analysis. *Lancet*, 383(9912), 166–175.
6. Chalmers I, Nylenna M (2014). A New Network to Promote Evidence-Based Research. *Lancet*, 384, 1903–1904.
7. Sheridan D (2013). *Advances in Medicine; How are they Made? In*: Medicak Science in the 21ˢᵗ Century; Sunset of New Dawn. London: Imperial College Press.
8. Barbour V (2003). UK Biobank: A Project in Search of a Protocol? *Lancet*, 361, 1734–1738.
9. Wallace H (2002). The Need for Independent Scientific Peer Review of Biobank UK. *Lancet*, 359, 2282.
10. Radda G, Dexter TM, Meade T (2002). The need for Independent Scientific Peer Review of Biobank UK; Reply from Biobank UK. *Lancet*, 359, 2282.
11. Millennium Seed Bank. Available at: http://www.kew.org/science-conservation/collections/millennium-seed-bank (Accessed on 8/12/2015).
12. http://en.wikipedia.org/wiki/John_Snow_%28physician%29 (Accessed on 8/12/2015).
13. Brody H, Russell Rip M, Vinten-Johansen P, Paneth N, Rachman S (1854). Map-making and Myth-making in Broad Street: The London Cholera Epidemic. *The Lancet*, 356.
14. Epidemiological Society (1854). *Lancet*, ii, 531.
15. Snow J (1854). The Cholera Near Golden-Square, and at Deptford. *Med Times Gazette*, 9, 321–322.
16. Snow J (2012). *On the Mode of Communication of Cholera*. London: John Churchill, New Burlington Street, England, 1855.
17. Tulodziecki D (2012). Principles of Reasoning in Historical Epidemiology. *J Eval Clin Pract*, 18, 968–973.
18. Gabbay J, Walley T (2006). Introducing New Health Interventions. *BMJ*, 332, 64–65.
19. Paneth N, Vinten-Johansen P, Brody H, Rip M (1998). A Rivalry of Foulness: Official and Unofficial Investigations of the London Cholera Epidemic of 1854. *Am J Public Health*, 88, 1545–1553.
20. Hemper S (2013). John Snow. *Lancet*, 381, 1269–1270.
21. Snow SJ (2008). John Snow: The Making of a Hero? *Lancet*, 372, 22–23.
22. Fleming A. Penicillin Nobel Lecture, December 11,1945. Available at: http://www.nobelprize.org/nobel_prizes/medicine/laureates/1945/fleming-lecture.pdf (Accessed on 8/12/2015).
23. Florey HW. Penicillin Nobel Lecture, December 11, 1945. Available at: http://www.nobelprize.org/nobel_prizes/medicine/laureates/1945/florey-lecture.pdf (Accessed on 8/12/2015).

24. The White House Press Secretary. President's 2016 Budget Proposes Historic Investment to Combat Antibiotic-Resistant Bacteria to Protect Public Health. Available at: https://www.whitehouse.gov/the-press-office/2015/01/27/fact-sheet-president-s-2016-budget-proposes-historic-investment-combat-a (Accessed on 8/12/2015).

25. Antimicrobial Resistance: Tackling a Crisis for the Health and Wealth of Nations. Available at: http://amr-review.org/ (Accessed on 8/12/2015).

26. Geoghegan-Quinn M (2014). Funding for Antimicrobial Resistance Research in Europe. *Lancet*, 384, 2186.

27. Lederberg J (2000). Infectious History. *Science*, 288, 287–293.

28. President's Council of Advisors on Science and Technology. Combating Antibiotic Resistance Sept 2014. Available at: https://www.whitehouse.gov/sites/default/files/microsites/ostp/PCAST/pcast_carb_report_sept2014.pdf (Accessed on 8/12/2015).

29. Department of Health, Department of Environment and Rural Affairs. UK Five Year Antimicrobial Resistance Strategy 2013 to 2018. Available at:: https://www.gov.uk/government/uploads/system/uploads/attachment_data/file/244058/20130902_UK_5_year_AMR_strategy.pdf (Accessed on 8/12/2015).

30. Gulliford MC, Dregan A, Moore MV, Ashworth M, van Staa T, McCann G, Charlton J, Yardley L, Little P, McDermott L (2014). Continued High Rates of Antibiotic Prescribing to Adults with Respiratory Tract Infection: Survey of 568 UK general practices. *BMJ Open*, 4:e006245.

31. Fleming A (1915). Some Notes on the Bacteriology of Gas Gangrene. *Lancet*, 186, 376–379.

32. Fleming A (1922). On a Remarkable Bacteriolytic Element Found in Tissues and Secretions. *Proc R Soc B*, 93(653), 306–317.

33. Fleming A (1929). On the Antibacterial Action of Cultures of a Penicillium, with Special Reference to Their Use in the Isolation of B. influenzae. *Br J Exp Pathol*, 10, 226–236. [Reprinted in Clinical Infectious diseases Vol. 2, No. 1 January–February 1980].

34. Chain E, Florey HW, Gardner AD, Heatley NG, Jennings MA, Orr-Ewing J, Sanders AG (1940). Penicillin as a Therapeutic Agent. *Lancet*, 236, 226–228.

35. Chain E. The Chemical Structure of the Penicillins. Nobel Lecture, March 20, 1946. Available at: http://www.nobelprize.org/nobel_prizes/medicine/laureates/1945/chain-lecture.pdf (Accessed on 8/12/2015).

36. House of Commons Science and Technology Committee, first report 2014–15. Ensuring access to working antimicrobials. Available at: http://www.publications.parliament.uk/pa/cm201415/cmselect/cmsctech/509/509.pdf (Accessed on 8/12/2015).

37. Sheridan DJ (2012). *The Decline of Biomedical Science Despite Unprecedented Technological Advances*: A 21st Century Paradox. *In*: Medical Science in the 21st Century; Sunset or New Dawn? London: Imperial College Press.

38. The World University Rankings 2013–2014. Available at: http://www.timeshighereducation.co.uk/world-university-rankings/2013-14/subject-ranking/subject/life-sciences (Accessed on 8/12/2015).

39. UK life sciences hit 7-year high Financial Times. Available at: http://www.ft.com/cms/s/0/6d0c13d6-4d55-11e4-bf60-00144feab7de.html#axzz3WcPyixRP (Accessed on 8/12/2015).

40. Horne B, Bell JI, ORavn MO, Tooke JE (2015). A New Social Contract for Medical Innovation. *Lancet*, 385, 1153–1154.

41. Doshi P (2015). Speeding New Antibiotics to Market: A Fake Fix? *BMJ*, 350, 17–19.

42. Sheridan DJ (2012). *Changes in medical professionalism in the 21st Century and their impact on medical science*. *In*: Medical Science in the 21st Century; Sunset or New Dawn? London: Imperial College Press.

Chapter 7

Impact of Evidence-Based Medicine on Clinical Practice: Achievements and Limitations

"He who studies medicine without books sails an uncharted sea,
but he who studies medicine without patients does not go to sea at all."

Sir William Osler

It seems to me that Osler's comment above embodies the idea of Evidence-Based Medicine (EBM). In referring to "books" Osler had in mind the principle of seeking knowledge based on written evidence from past experience which may assist in caring for patients. He emphasises the importance of looking beyond the knowledge and experience which is immediately available. However, his metaphor goes further than that by stressing that crucial evidence is derived from the clinical interaction with patients. In this he differed from the version of EBM advocated in recent times, which stressed the value of published evidence from clinical trials as greater than clinical evidence or experience. We now recognise that all written evidence is not equal and that the expansion of medical research during 20th century and especially the development of randomised controlled trials require us to pay particular attention to the quality of evidence on which written evidence is based. The EBM movement succeeded in bringing this to the attention of medicine and indeed the wider public in its remarkable rhetorical campaign in the early 1990s. Osler's comment might be criticised for failing to distinguish and prioritise which books provide the best evidence, which the EBM movement did very well. However, this would seem to miss his central point, the need to seek evidence from a wide range of sources. Future generations may come to look on Osler's comment as wiser for two reasons. First, a century ago it would not have been possible to predict what forms of medical evidence would emerge and this also holds true now. The idea that we can set down in perpetuity even the best randomised controlled trials as the supreme form of medical evidence seems unwise. Second, as I write there is increasing concern that an over-emphasis on "data" from clinical trials and systematic reviews at the expense of clinical evidence risks marginalising the patients' concerns and obscuring their humanity and dignity.[1]

EBM: Impact of Medicine

Medicine has undergone many changes in its history. In recent memory, however, no other movement has succeeded in capturing the agenda for deciding the future of clinical practice more effectively than EBM (Box 7.1). Its presence is felt almost universally in healthcare; we read of it weekly in the literature; there are at least five journals devoted to EBM and another half dozen using "evidence-based" as a suffix to a specialty interest for example evidence-based nursing. There is a website for it. We have academic departments of EBM, Centres of EBM and professorships of EBM. We now find the brand "evidence-based" extended to other activities as in "evidence-based decision making" and "evidence-based research". It is difficult to think of any other health related campaign which has been more successful than the EBM movement, other than perhaps the efforts to raise awareness and funding to combat AIDs and some famine relief campaigns. However, even these were focused on single issues and limited in time. In contrast, EBM has grown and extended its influence over more than two decades.

The Cochrane Collaboration is the single most prominent achievement of EBM. As discussed in Chapter 3, it provides each year over 400 systematic reviews of clinical trials related to treatments over a wide range of medical specialties. Over the years, these have accumulated into a solid body of work which enables health workers, scientists, commissioners and policy makers to access summaries of work to date in a wide range of fields. Its success in recruiting over 40,000 volunteers around the world to undertake this work

---

Box 7.1   Impact of the EBM: Achievements.

1. The most successful health campaign in recent medical history.
2. Timely recognition and response to emerging health priorities.
3. Development of the Cochrane Collaboration.
4. Harnessing over 40,000 volunteers world-wide to support its mission.
5. Advocating the need for evidence of efficacy and cost effectiveness in assessing new therapies.
6. Contributing to the development of clinical guidelines.
7. Advocating the need for full disclosure of clinical trial data.
8. Contributing to awareness of overdiagnosis.

---

is a good measure of its popularity and success. The creation of the Cochrane Library to maintain and make available its systematic reviews was a further major development, and has been highly successful as indicated by almost 4 million full-text downloads in 2010. The library has also begun to generate significant income to support its work, providing about 6% of its funding in 2009. These are remarkable achievements by any standard. The reasons for its success are several. Most importantly, the group which initiated and maintain the movement has shown extraordinary commitment and dedication to the project from the outset and this has not wavered with time. It has been well organised as a group and has maintained its coherence with regular meetings over the years. One of its founders likened the group's belief in its mission and its intensity and commitment to that of Jesuit priests, as if "signed up for life".

Two aspects of its methods stand out in explaining its success. First, its rise to prominence reflects a highly skilful use of rhetoric. The phrase "EBM" was a stroke of genius. Who could be opposed to it? Who would support non-EBM? It not only helped to disarm any possible opposition but also promised something that everybody would want. And indeed everyone did seem to want it as evident by its wide adoption in headlines among the general media[2–5]; it could be said to have gone "viral" in the days before e-media were ready for it. Importantly it also claimed the moral high ground for the group and its ideas. A second feature of the group's success has been its commitment to maintaining its presence and mission in media and literature. As would be expected, a high proportion of the publications by leading members' of the group are systematic reviews (25% of the total). However, their publication of editorials and opinion pieces was more than double that, which is exceptional in medicine or medical science and would be inconceivable for most clinicians and scientists. It indicates a powerful commitment to advocacy which the group has maintained and this too has been an important reason for its success.

A further factor which contributed to the success of EBM was its timeliness. During the late 20th century, delivering healthcare emerged as a major political and economic issue for most western counties due to rising costs and demand. As a result, interest in ways to improve efficiency, outcomes and quality of care increased sharply among health care managers and policy makers. Around this time, also as discussed in Chapter 4, a major shift in the control of funding for medical science occurred particularly in the UK. For most of the 20th century, the dominant view had been that science in general is best led by scientists. This was challenged by Lord Rothschild in 1972, whose report led to the introduction of the purchaser–provider concept whereby funders of research would commission it to meet its needs. This failed and was later substantially reversed in 1981. However, Rothschild's ideas were later reintroduced following a parliamentary committee enquiry into medical research in 1988, and as a result a substantial proportion of funding for medical research came under the direct control the Department of Health. This in turn shifted interest in research towards more practical health care delivery needs, and away from exploratory science. This led to the birth of what became known as "health related research". The ideas of EBM promising more cost effective and improved care would have been ideally suited to this. Some might say that the timing of EBM was fortuitous; however, that may be underestimating the foresight and strategy of the leaders of the movement. In any event, the growth of EBM and the founding of the Cochrane Collaboration benefitted from a political back drop which made funding available for research into improving the efficiency of delivering healthcare.

Clinical Guidelines

At the time EBM was launched there was growing interest in the use of clinical guidelines as a means to improve clinical practice by bringing the most recent up to date research to bear on clinical decision-making and thereby to improve efficiency.[6] Indeed, some guidelines had already appeared.[7] Guidelines would provide systematically developed statements about care for specific conditions to assist clinicians' and patients' decisions.[8] At this time too, attempts were being made to introduce an element of market economics into healthcare in the UK and guidelines were proposed as a means to assist this by providing purchasers and providers with information on which to build contracts.[9] Over the past two decades, a veritable industry has grown around providing such guidelines involving a large number of organisations. In the UK, guidelines are produced by the National Institute for Clinical Excellence (NICE), The Scottish Intercollegiate Guidelines Network, The Guidelines and Audit Implementation Network as well as Professional Organisations and Royal Colleges. NICE began producing guidelines around 2000 and this had increased four-fold by 2004. At the time of writing, NICE maintains a database of 229 guidelines with 97 in development.[10] There is considerable cooperation among the various bodies undertaking guideline production in the UK and most of the effort is coordinated through NICE. In addition, guidelines are produced by international professional societies, for example in my own specialty The European Society of Cardiology has produced 32 clinical guidelines,[11] which are endorsed by its member national societies and therefore will also influence practice locally. The numbers quoted above do not reflect the overall volume of guidelines produced or their impact. One small survey of guidelines in clinical practice examined the applicability of guidelines to patients admitted during an acute medical intake in which 18 patients were seen among whom 44 diagnosis were made. The published guidelines relevant to these amounted to 3,679 document pages and even this was limited to guidelines published during the preceding 3 years by the main producers.[12] In order to be up to date with these would have taken an estimated 122 hours of reading time. Clinical guidelines are intimately related to EBM because they provide the means to disseminate the evidence which the EBM movement sought to bring to bear on practice; in effect they became the primary means to implement EBM. In addition, since the production of clinical guidelines depends on evaluating published research including systematic reviews, the work of the Cochrane Collaboration has made a major contribution to their production.

National Institute for Clinical Excellence (NICE)

Clinical guidance produced by NICE in particular has grown to play a major role in medicine, both in the UK and internationally. Founded in 2000 as an integral part of the NHS, it foresaw the need to maintain its independence in developing its guidance from both government and from the pharmaceutical industry. In its early days, concerns that it would be a mechanism for rationing health services were refuted vigorously[13] by its first chairman who recognised at the outset that unless it earned the respect of public opinion it would fail in its mission to be an independent standards setting body. Initially, its role was to evaluate the effectiveness of new therapies and devices, and this was extended later to include an element of cost effectiveness known as health technology assessment. In order to measure cost effectiveness comprehensively, it was recognised that the efficacy of therapies needed to be assessed not just in terms of lives saved, but also by a measure of their ability to improve the quality of life. This led to the introduction of what is known as quality adjusted life years (QALY), meaning that one year lived in perfect health carries a QALY value of 1. The QALY value declines towards 0 as the degree of disability increases. Measured in this way drugs are required to deliver an improved quality of life at a cost which is lower than a set cash threshold of £20000–£30000 per QALY. Although this has resulted in a number of controversial decisions and stimulated further research on what an acceptable threshold should be,[14] it has become accepted as a means to assess cost effectiveness. For patient groups hoping for better treatments, decisions to decline funding can be very disappointing and in some cases has led to political debate and in the case of cancer drugs, to some adjustment of the threshold.[15] Pharmaceutical companies too were concerned that cost effectiveness evaluations by NICE would represent a major new challenge for their products. That however, appears to have subsided substantially and there is now a general acceptance that economic evaluation of new drugs and devices is a reality and here to stay and not just in the UK. Similar organisations have now been developed in many countries.[16] By 2005, NICE had received visits from representatives from 60 countries and had almost 60,000 hits on its website from overseas everyday.[17] The work of NICE and similar organisations around the world represents a major change in medicine and the advocacy of the EBM movement can rightly claim significant credit for changing the public and political atmosphere which made this possible, and it continues to play an important role in the evaluations undertaken by NICE and other organisations through its work in evaluating research evidence.

Impact of Guidelines in Clinical Practice

Guidelines are now an everyday part of clinical practice and have become an important element of clinical and patient decisions. To what extent have they changed the way those decisions are made and what effect has this had on patient care? One early review of studies which examined the impact of guidelines showed evidence of changes in practice in the direction indicated by the guidelines.[9] Most of these studies were limited to measuring the impact on clinical practice; only 11 of 59 studies examined the effect on patient outcomes. Of these, almost all showed some benefit. Researchers have been mostly interested in exploring how best to disseminate guidelines in order to effect doctors' compliance with them. Important factors which influence doctors' adherence to guidelines relate to their source: in particular those originating from well known, authoritative and respected organisations such as NICE having greater impact.[18–20] In addition, high level policy decisions on health priorities were important. Later studies suggested that as the number of guidelines being produced increased, their source and quality became more variable. Thus by 2008, general practitioners were concerned that some guidelines were not based on reliable evidence and were of little value. Others were concerned that some producers of guidelines were unaware of conditions in general practice; for example, a requirement for patients with heart failure to have echocardiograms when the equipment was not available. For most doctors, guidelines which are backed by respected authoritative figures are likely to have much greater impact.[21] The growing number of guidelines also meant that it became harder to bring them to the attention of clinicians and further efforts were needed to do so. Making guidelines available on-line has been studied as a possible means to do this. However, the results again appear to be variable. As in previous studies, the means of delivering guidelines appears to be less important than that they represent a consensus view and are promoted by trusted knowledgeable sources.[22] Guidelines also vary depending on whether they are derived from local or national sources.[23] Furthermore, as guidelines are increasingly produced in different countries the emphasis and focus they bring to clinical situations can differ.

For example, a review of guidelines for pain recognition and management in palliative care in 11 European countries showed marked differences.[24] Similar findings of variable implementation were revealed by studies of guidelines in several European countries; however, once again uptake appears to depend heavily on the source of guidelines, whether they are supported by a consensus and have the backing of respected organisations.[25-27] After more than two decades of intense interest and a major research effort resulting in a large number of publications, reliable data on what impact clinical guidelines have had on patient care is quite poor. Initial hopes[28] have not materialised and early evidence of benefit has not been reliably confirmed.[9] Part of the reason for this is the sheer volume of guidelines now being produced. Coordination of guideline production through NICE by specialist societies and the Royal Colleges appears to be most effective in gaining traction among physicians. There seems little doubt that clinical guidelines produced from such sources have significant impact and are here to stay. Although clinical guidelines were already emerging when the EBM movement launched its campaign, its advocacy of clinical trial evidence and later systematic reviews were an important contribution to their recognition and expansion and in time this may prove to be one of the most important contributions of EBM.

Wider Impact of EBM

Advocacy and lobbying have a useful role in society in focusing attention on particular injustices, inequities or other deficiencies. This is also the case in health care and there have been several recent successful campaigns in highlighting, for example, the plight of people suffering from AIDs and famine. In any such campaign, inevitably there has to be a focus and determination to carry it forward. The EBM movement has shown remarkable success in this and its focus on evidence has led to a greater awareness not just of published evidence, but on evidence which may be missing from the literature and on published evidence which may be unreliable.

Full Disclosure of Clinical Trials

As discussed in Chapter 3, members of the Cochrane Collaboration led a major campaign against Hoofman–LaRoche and GlaxoSmithKline for full disclosure of clinical trial data in relation to the anti-flu drugs zanamivir and oseltamivir which was eventually successful. The case arose because systematic reviews of clinical trials may be unreliable if full information is not available. In doing so, the case contributed to a much wider recognition of the need for full disclosure of clinical research undertaken by the pharmaceutical industry, culminating in calls for prompt reporting and full disclosure of clinical trials by World Health Organisation[29] and the European Union.[30]

Overdiagnosis in Medicine

The challenge of overdiagnosing medical conditions has been recognised for several decades. However, of 448 articles found in PubMed since 1973, 424 were published since 1990 and 380 since 2000 indicating a growing awareness of the problem. The issue now arises in almost every medical specialty, but has been of particular concern in relation to screening for breast cancer and prostate cancer. The issue is best exemplified by dramatic increases in the diagnosis of certain conditions during the past three decades for which mortality rates have hardly changed. Thus, diagnosis of new cases of thyroid cancer doubled between 1975 and 2005 in the US, while deaths from it were unchanged; similarly, cases of melanoma increased three fold with no change in mortality from it. The same pattern has been observed for kidney, breast and prostate cancer.[31] Some of this will be the result of earlier and better treatment, but a substantial amount of it reflects disease which would never have caused symptoms. This is known because many cancers progress so slowly that they are only known about when found fortuitously at post mortem in people who have died from other causes. The most striking example of this is prostate cancer. Careful studies of prostate glands at post-mortem in men who died from accidents showed a striking increase in cancer with age. It was detected in around 70% of men over the age of 60 and around 80% in those over 70 years.[32] This substantial reservoir means that if tests had been carried out while they were alive, a significant number would have been diagnosed and treated with no benefit and the likelihood being that some would have been harmed.

The concern then is that tests may reveal a suspected diagnosis, for example, of prostate cancer after finding an elevated Prostate Specific Antigen (PSA) level leading to further investigations and possible treatment including surgery. This raises two possible problems. First, some patients will inevitably experience some complications related to these interventions and second prostate cancer in some cases is well known to progress very slowly over decades and many people who develop it never experience any symptoms of disability from it. Consequently, although well intentioned, the diagnosis and treatment of prostate cancer may be harming some people. Similar concerns have been raised about screening for breast cancer and many other investigations in healthy people. It also impacts on health services more widely because of the costs involved, and this will undoubtedly keep it firmly on the health agenda for the foreseeable future, given the pressures facing health services due to increasing demand and costs. As I write, new campaigns to limit overdiagnosis and overtreatment seem to reflect this.[33,34]

However, the problem of overdiagnosis is also raising concerns in that it reflects changes in attitudes among patients and clinicians.[35] As discussed in Chapter 5, all clinical encounters between patients and clinicians begin with uncertainty; the aim being to reduce it as far as possible in reaching a diagnosis. However, some degree of residual uncertainty is always unavoidable. Some argue that doctors' willingness to accept this in managing patients has decreased in recent years for a variety of reasons including fears that they may be criticised for making errors or even worse, suspended or punished if things go wrong. The natural consequence is to act defensively to ensure that no stone is left unturned, resulting in more tests and investigations. In addition, many people hearing advice about healthy life styles and the risks they need to avoid are also made more aware of potential illnesses they may encounter and this coupled with the reality of our finite lives also serves to increase their fears. Doctors may also be more inclined to carry out tests in the hope of allaying the fears of worried patients leading to a cycle of increased medical interventions. Two other factors may also contribute to this. Variations in the incidence of cancer rates between populations and countries have increased interest in prevention and diagnosis. For example, even in the UK, Scotland has a 15% higher rate of cancer mortality than the UK as a whole.[36] In addition, cancer survival rates vary between countries, the UK having survival rates below the European average for most common cancers.[37] Inevitably this emphasises the need for earlier and better detection rates and in turn to the increased use of tests, which may also increase the detection rate of some cancers which otherwise might never have caused symptoms, and so to overdiagnosis and treatment. Furthermore, the increased use of guidelines and rule-following based on data, coupled with a greater use of appraisal based on them, relegates clinical judgement and contributes to a culture in which doing tests may be considered "safer" than doing nothing. The advocacy of the EBM movement may have contributed to this as an unintended consequence of its emphasis on data and rule following. It is also paradoxical of course since overdiagnosis is in reality an example of incorrect diagnosis and therefore of non-EBM.

In addition, prevention of ill health due to harmful lifestyles is increasingly important but cannot be promoted without raising awareness of disease. But as populations are advised to lead healthy lifestyles they also become more aware of potential illnesses they may encounter, which may also increase their anxiety and fears. Furthermore, extension of what is abnormal also expands the population needing treatment. For example, lowering of thresholds for risk factors such as hypertension increases the number of people needing treatment. Some regard this as aggressive tactics by pharmaceutical companies seeking to increase their markets and to the unnecessary medicalising of normal people.[38] It seems to me that overdiagnosis and over treatment is framing up to become a major issue in medicine during the years ahead. Recognition of the problem has much to do with EBM, and is another example of the impact of the EBM movement has had on health care.

EBM: Unintended Consequences

The strength of the EBM movement has been a reflection of the focus of its mission and its determination to pursue it. But like all campaigns the need to focus on a restricted agenda can lead to unforeseen consequences in areas not covered by its mission (Box 7.2). This is not unusual and was seen for example in the AIDs campaign which proved highly successful in making anti-viral drugs available for millions of people around the world, but failed adequately to address the means of how to deliver them and distracted attention from other needs, some of which were a cause of even greater mortality.[39] Needs and priorities change with time and movements may need to adapt to remain relevant. In the case of EBM there are increasing concerns that it too may have had unintended consequences and needs to change. Some go so far as to describe the movement as being in crisis.[1]

Box 7.2   Impact of the EBM: Limitations.

1. A restricted view of evidence needed to practice clinical medicine.
2. Poor representation and lack of clinical expertise among its members.
3. An over emphasis on collective data at the expense of individual patient needs.
4. Failure to recognise the importance and value of the clinical encounter.
5. Imposition of methods of population medicine on clinical practice.
6. An over emphasis on data contributing to a bias in favour of what is easily measurable.

What Evidence?

Evidence derived from published research is just one element of knowledge required by doctors and patients to make clinical decisions. However, it is the single most important aspect on which the concept of EBM is based and the purpose of most of the work of the movement. The published evidence which is available therefore is crucial to its mission. In recent years, concerns have been raised that much of what is published may in fact be false resulting in confusion and wasted resources.[40] As discussed in Chapter 3, it has been argued that 85% of research funding is wasted. There are also concerns that drug companies seeking to meet regulatory and cost effectiveness requirements may be gaming their research designs by choosing comparators and doses in order to advantage their products.[41] Trials may also be designed using very large study populations in order to show statistical significance for minor therapeutic effects.[42] All of this is claimed to be distorting the EBM "brand",[11] and to undermine science. From the point of view of EBM, however, exposing research weaknesses and seeking ways to improve them could be thought of as part of its mission. After all, if EBM is to have value it must be based on reliable evidence and if statistical standards are unreliable in research, then improving them is an essential prerequisite for EBM to be meaningful and can only be beneficial for medicine.

Value of Evidence and Evidence of Value

The value of any evidence can be seen to relate to its accuracy and proximity to the truth. But in another sense the value of evidence relates to its worth in a much wider sense. Evidence which leads to a better understanding of something, to an improvement in human well being or to better management of the environment for example, might have no immediate utility value related to the purpose of the research which produced it. How should the value of such evidence then be measured? Would an analysis of the statistical methods used in the research which led to it provide a measure of its value? If it turned out that there were weaknesses in the study design would they diminish the value of the knowledge gained? Alexander Fleming's initial observation that penicillium mould produced a substance which destroyed *staphylococci* was based on a single observation, as discussed in Chapter 6. What was its value? If measured purely in statistical terms it had no value. However, its potential value in a wider sense was great as Fleming suspected. In order to prove that his suspicions were correct Fleming needed to undertake a formal study. However, this included no formal statistical analysis.[43] What then was the value of his research? Clearly, it had immense value as was recognised by Fleming sharing the Noble Prize. But if included in an assessment of the value of science based on the statistical procedures used in research, it would have fared badly. It would of course be nonsense to suggest that reliable statistical methods are unimportant in research. However, it is equally invalid to claim that statistical precision alone can be used to determine the value of research or that research which fails to meet statistical criteria is necessarily unreliable or wasteful.

For EBM, the value of evidence is mostly concerned with the analysis of clinical trials which are undertaken to assess the safety and efficacy of treatments to meet regulatory requirements. They use broadly standard designs and statistical analysis and to that extent the quality of their design and methods can provide a measure of their reliability. Furthermore, they require human participation which is not without risk. Consequently, there is a particular responsibility that they should be carried out to the highest standard. In contrast, most original science is exploratory and undertaken to uncover new knowledge. Exploring novel questions requires methods which may need to be designed specifically to test the hypotheses being studied. Their methods therefore are less comparable across a range of experiments. Statistical methods are still important but are less useful as a single measure of reliability and value. In addition, it is expected that findings of some original science will be refuted by later studies and this is regarded as part of the growth of knowledge. When Newton's understanding of gravity was overturned by Einstein's theory of relativity in the 20th century, it was a cause of celebration; there was no sense that Newton's work had failed or was wasteful. Therefore, the idea that all research can be valued or condemned as wasteful on the basis of the statistical methods used is not reliable.

Bias of the Easily Measurable

EBM has done much to bring the most reliable published evidence to bear on medical practice and to the development of clinical guidelines based on it. It brought a much needed objectivity and measurable dimension with its emphasis on published trial data. Clinical guidelines can also provide a basis on which to compare performance and cost efficiency. In doing so, EBM has focused attention on a wide range of measurable outcomes. We can measure complication and mortality rates following surgery, length of stay in hospitals for particular conditions, rates of acquired infections in hospitals and so on, all of which provide valuable insights about care. However, this data — analysis approach to medicine — also has limitations for several reasons. First, it is never possible to measure everything simultaneously in complex systems such as health care and what is chosen to measure may inadvertently impact areas not under scrutiny. For example, if it is known that performance in a particular area is being measured, shifting resources to support it temporarily may be used to enhance it, but could adversely affect other areas. Second, what may appear to be reliable measures of performance, as for example mortality and readmission rates for pneumonia can be manipulated either consciously or unconsciously.[44] And of course such measures of performance may provide little information about the experiences of individual patients. Attempting to measure performance in health care is clearly important. However, pressures to do so in efforts to improve cost efficiency or to demonstrate progress towards it can lead to an over reliance on what measures are available rather than suitable, and to a selection bias of the easily measurable.

Many clinicians and patients including supporters of EBM have raised concerns that the emphasis on collective and averaged data has distracted attention from the needs of individual patients[11] and that clinical guidelines can objectify patients as units requiring interventions rather than people needing empathy and dialogue in making decisions about their care.[45] Disputes between public health experts concerned about reducing the burden of illness in populations, and general practitioners concerned about treating individual patients is another reflection of this. Averaged data may indicate that treating groups of people will reduce the burden of illness in the population, but it cannot reveal whether some of them individually may be unsuitable to receive it or even by harmed by it. The controversy of the use of anti-viral drugs to treat healthy people as discussed in Chapter 3 illustrates this well; public health experts were keen to treat healthy people in the hope of reducing the burden of flu in the population, whereas general practitioners were concerned that side effects might be more harmful for some frail elderly people. There is a need for balance between managing the health of populations and of individuals; similarly, the drive for administrative efficiency in health care must not undermine the needs of individual patients. The priority given to trial data in EBM has been helpful in bringing the latest research to bear on clinical management, but its failure adequately to recognise the importance and value of clinical evidence derived from individual patients may have contributed to a culture in which the needs and dignity of patients were over ridden in favour of administrative efficiency resulting in neglect with serious consequences for many.[46]

"Real EBM" — A New Iteration of EBM?

Recently, it has been argued that EBM has gone astray and may be in crisis and needs reconfiguration. The language used is EBM being in crisis and needing to be replaced by "Real EBM".[11] The argument here is that EBM has been undermined by attempts to subvert it by vested interests seeking advantage, for example by pharmaceutical companies seeking to extend their markets by producing evidence of benefit using lower treatment thresholds for conditions such as hypertension, diabetes and cancer;[47] some of this evidence being statistically correct but biologically insignificant. There are also concerns that well intentioned efforts to improve the delivery of evidence-based care by automated computerised methods shift clinical consultations away from the needs and interests of individual patients towards the management of population groups. Consultations tend to become bureaucratic responses to the computer system rather than the purpose of the patient's concerns.[48] This is enhanced by the use of screen "pop-ups" to help direct the consultation in the direction predetermined by EBM but in practice serves to further distract both the carer and patient from the reasons for the patients visit. Such templates fail to take account of the reality that many patients and particularly the elderly are on treatment for other conditions not included in the particular template or guidelines being followed in pursuit of delivering EBM. And so "Real EBM" has been proposed which would put individual patients at the forefront of the clinical encounter. Rule following would give way to expert judgements and care would be provided in the context of professional relationships between clinicians and patients based on continuity and empathy.[11] The best research evidence would still have an important role but would be practiced around the individual patient's need and experience, recognising that for some patients it could be inappropriate or even perverse, for example those who are terminally ill. I suggest that most clinicians would endorse these views and patients too would welcome a system which recognises them as individuals and respects their experience and dignity. But is this "Real EBM" or simply medicine practiced in a professional and responsible manner? Do we really need a new brand, a new movement and new rhetoric to reinvent what Osler was reminding us of a century ago? EBM has done much good in emphasising the importance of research evidence in medicine, but as advocated it also had inherent weaknesses which have contributed to the difficulties clinicians and patients now experience. These relate not only to the concepts advocated by the movement but also to its rhetorical methods.

The concept that medicine should be based on evidence is an obvious good, but from the outset, the EBM movement proclaimed a priority for evidence as data and argued for the relegation of the professional and clinical aspects of care which are now recognised as being in need of recovery. From the outset also the EBM movement lacked a strong clinical base, being composed mostly of epidemiologists, statisticians and public health interests and so it is hardly surprising that it failed adequately to recognise and preserve the individualised medicine now felt to be under threat. Its remarkable success in establishing its brand and advocating its ideas pushed the movement to the forefront of the healthcare agenda and convinced many that it is a new system for practicing medicine. Indeed, the sheer success of its advocacy has contributed to the cul-de-sac clinical medicine now finds itself in.[49] However, as Osler recognised, you have to experience the clinical encounter and have the training and aptitude to engage in it effectively in order to understand the importance and value of the patient experience. What has been so successfully branded as EBM is in reality, a system which generates summary research evidence in support of medical practice. Valuable though this is, it is not a method for caring for patients. The challenge therefore is to recognise and reclaim clinical medicine (in the broad sense including all aspects of patient care) as the professional activity which cares for patients. Clinical medicine is how this should be described, rather than rebranded EBM.

Conclusions

The concept of EBM has had a remarkable impact on medicine since it was launched in the early 1990s. It was founded at a time when reforms were being introduced in health care systems which were seeking ways to improve efficiency and cost effectiveness to manage rising costs and demands. Its founders proved to be highly effective advocates in capturing the health agenda, and in maintaining a coherent and well organised movement. The Cochrane Collaboration became a major aspect of its work and its success in attracting 40,000 volunteers world wide to maintain its commitment, to publish systematic reviews of published medical research is a good measure of its success. It has contributed to major changes in medicine mainly through the introduction of clinical guidelines and highlighting challenges such as over diagnosis. It continues to shine a light on weaknesses in our research systems by advocating the full disclosure of clinical trials.

Despite these achievements there is also a growing sense that the evidence-based movement has also had some adverse effects on clinical medicine, leading to claims that it is in crisis and needs to adapt. The principal concerns are that the movement overemphasised the importance of published data at the expense of clinical evidence, and as a result contributed to undermining the encounter between patients and clinicians. As a result, it is argued that the empathic and ethical basis of clinical medicine has suffered and the needs and experience of patients have been marginalised. From the beginning, the evidence-based movement has lacked adequate representation of clinical experience, being largely composed of epidemiologists, statisticians and public health interests and this may have contributed to a tendency to impose methods suitable for population medicine on clinical practice. This has also arisen in part because of the misleading claim implicit in the title EBM, which led many to believe that it is a system for the care of patients. In reality, it is a movement which advocates the use of published evidence in medicine and contributes to the production of synthesised summaries of published research. These have been broadly welcomed by and supported by clinical medicine, however, it is now argued that individual patient care needs to be restored so that the interests and dignity of patients is fully acknowledged and respected. This cannot be achieved simply by a rebranding of EBM; instead, it will require clinical medicine to reclaim its role as the proper means to care for individual patients based on its professional and ethical values and responsibilities.

References

1. Greenhalgh T, Howick J, Maskrey N (2014). Evidence Based Medicine: A Movement in Crisis? *BMJ*, 348, g3725.
2. The Year in Ideas: A to Z.; Evidence-Based Medicine New York Times Magazine. Dec 9th 2001. Available at: http://www.nytimes.com/2001/12/09/magazine/the-year-in-ideas-a-to-z-evidence-based-medicine.html (Accessed on 9/12/2015).
3. Are Doctors just Playing Hunches? Time Magazine. Available at: http://content.time.com/time/magazine/article/0,9171,1590448,00.html (Accessed on 9/12/2015).
4. In Praise of Anecdotal Evidence, The Guardian. Available at: http://www.theguardian.com/healthcare-network/2012/sep/03/in-praise-of-anecdotal-evidence (Accessed on 9/12/2015).
5. Pediatrician Advocates Use of 'Evidence-Based Medicine' in Japan. The Japan Times. Available at: http://www.japantimes.co.jp/news/2015/01/05/national/science-health/pediatrician-advocates-use-evidence-based-medicine-japan/ (Accessed on 9/12/2015).
6. Irning D (1991). *Managing Quality in General Practice*. London: King's Fund.
7. British Thoracic Society (1990). Guidelines for Management of Asthma in Adults: I — Chronic Persistent Asthma. *BMJ*, 301, 651–653.
8. Institute of Medicine (1992). *Guidelines for Clinical Practice: From Development to Use*. Washington, DC: National Academic Press.
9. Grimshaw J, Russell I (1993). Achieving Health Gain Through Clinical Guidelines. I: Developing Scientifically Valid Guidelines. *Qual Health Care*, 2, 243–248.
10. National Institute for Clinical Excellence; Guidance List. Available at: http://www.nice.org.uk/guidance/published?type=guidelines (Accessed on 9/12/2015).
11. European Society of Cardiology, Clinical Practice Guidelines. Available at: http://www.escardio.org/Guidelines-&-Education/Clinical-Practice-Guidelines/listing (Accessed on 9/12/2015).

12. Allen D, Harkins K (2005). Too Much Guidance? *Lancet*, 365, 1768.

13. Rawlins M. House of Commons — Select Committee on Health Minutes of Evidence. Available at: parliament.uk.http://www.publications.parliament.uk/pa/cm199899/cmselect/cmhealth/222/9020406.htm (Accessed on 9/12/2015).

14. Woods B, Revill P, Sculpher M, Claxton K. Country-level Cost-Effectiveness Thresholds: Initial Estimates and the Need for Further Research. Available at: http://www.york.ac.uk/media/che/documents/papers/researchpapers/CHERP109_cost-effectiveness_threshold_LMICs.pdf (Accessed on 9/12/2015).

15. Dyer C (2009). Health Department Sets up Cost Sharing Deal for Multiple Myeloma Drug. *BMJ*, 338, b423.

16. Marcial VG, Juan ABA, Americo C, Davide I, Inger NN, Beatriz V, Annette Z. *Health Technology Assessment in Europe — Overview of the Producers. In*: Health Technology Assessment and Health Policy-Making in Europe Current Status, Challenges and Potential. Available at: http://www.euro.who.int/en/health-topics/Health-systems/health-technologies (Accessed on 9/12/2015).

17. Rawlins MD (2005). 5 NICE years. *Lancet*, 365, 904–908.

18. Harrison S, Dowswell G, Wright J, Russell I (2003). General Practitioners' Uptake of Clinical Practice Guidelines: A Qualitative Study. *J Health Serv Res Policy*, 8(3), 149–153.

19. Wroblewski BM, Siney PD, Fleming PA (2003). Wear of Enhanced Ultra-high Molecular-weight Polyethylene (Hylamer) in Combination with a 22.225 mm Diameter Zirconia Femoral Head. *J Bone Joint Surg [Br]*, 85-B, 376–379.

20. Westcott K, Irvine GH (2002). Appropriateness of Referrals for Removal of Wisdom Teeth. *Brit J Oral Max Surg*, 40, 304–306.

21. Rashidian A, Eccles MP, Russell I, (2008). Falling on Stony Ground? A Qualitative Study of Implementation of Clinical Guidelines' Prescribing Recommendations in Primary Care. *Health Policy*, 85, 148–161.

22. Williams JG, Cheung WY, Price DE, Tansey R, Russell IT, Duane PD, Al-Ismail SA, Wani MA (2004). Clinical Guidelines Online: Do They Improve Compliance? *Postgrad Med J*, 80, 415–419.

23. Jokhan S, Whitworth MK, Jones F, Saunders A, Heazell AEP (2015). Evaluation of the Quality of Guidelines for the Management of Reduced Fetal Movements in UK Maternity units. *BMC Preg Childbirth*, 15, 54.

24. Sampson EL, van der Steen JT, Pautex S, Svartzman P, Sacchi V, Van den Block L, Van Den Noortgate N (2015). European Palliative Care Guidelines: How Well do They Meet the Needs of People with Impaired Cognition? *BMJ S P Care*, pii, bmjspcare-2014-000813.

25. Sandström B, Willman A, Svensson B, Borglin G (2015). Perceptions of National Guidelines and their (non) Implementation in Mental Healthcare: A Deductive and Inductive Content Analysis. *Implement Sci*, 10, 43.

26. Nowakowski A, Cybulski M, Śliwczyński A, Chil A, Teter Z, Seroczyński P, Arbyn M, Anttila A (2015). The Implementation of an Organised Cervical Screening Programme in Poland: An Analysis of the Adherence to European Guidelines. *BMC*, 15, 279.

27. O'Higgins A, Dunne F, Lee B, Smith D, Turner MJ. A National Survey of Implementation of Guidelines for Gestational Diabetes Mellitus Abstract: UCD Centre for Human Reproduction, Coombe Women.

28. Grimshaw JM, Hutchinson A (1995, 2014). Clinical Practice Guidelines — Do they Enhance Value for Money in Health Care? Br M Bulle, 51, 927. *Ir Med J*, 107(8), 231–233.

29. Moorthy VS, Karam G, Vannice KS, Kieny M_P. Rationale for WHO's New Position Calling for Prompt Reporting and Public Disclosure of Interventional Clinical Trial Results. *PLoS Med* 12(4), e1001819.

30. EU's Clinical Trials Regulation "A Step in Right Direction". Available at: https://www.theparliamentmagazine.eu/articles/sponsored_article/pm-eu%E2%80%99s-clinical-trials-regulation-%E2%80%98-step-right-direction%E2%80%99 (Accessed on 9/12/2015).

31. Gilbert WH, Black WC (2010). Overdiagnosis in Cancer. *JNCI*, 102, 605–613.

32. Sakr WA, Grignon DJ, Haas GP, Heilbrun LK, Pontes JE, Crissman JD (1996). Age and Racial Distribution of Prostatic Intraepithelial Neoplasia. *Eur Urol*, 30(2), 138–144.

33. Too Much Medicine. Available at: http://www.bmj.com/too-much-medicine. (Accessed on 9/12/2015).

34. Preventing Overdiagnosis. Available at: http://www.preventingoverdiagnosis.net.

35. Heath I. (2014). Role of Fear in Overdiagnosis and Overtreatment. *BMJ*, 349, g6123.

36. Cancer Incidence and Mortality in the UK (2008–2010). Office of National Statistics. Available at: http://www.ons.gov.uk/ons/rel/cancer-unit/cancer-incidence-and-mortality/2008-2010/stb-cancer-incidence-and-mortality-in-the-united-kindom--2008-2010.html (Accessed on 1/5/2015).

37. De Angelis R, Sant M, Coleman MP *et al.* and the EUROCARE-5 Working Group (2014). Cancer survival in Europe 1999–2007 by Country and Age: Results of EUROCARE-5 — A Population-Based Study. *Lancet Oncol*, 15, 23–34.

38. Feinstein AR, Sosin DM, Wells CK (1985). The Will Rogers Phenomenon. Stage Migration and New Diagnostic Techniques as a Source of Misleading Statistics for Survival in Cancer. *N Engl J Med*, 312, 1604–1608.

39. Sheridan D (2012). *The Impact of the Changing Social, Political and Economic Environment on Medical Science. In*: Medical Science in the 21st Century: Sunset or New Dawn. London: Imperial College Press.

40. Ioannidis JPA (2005). Why Most Published Research Findings are False. *PLoS Med*, 2(8), e124.

41. Heres S, Davis J, Maino K, Jetzinger E, Kissling W, Leucht S (2006). Why Olanzapine Beats Risperidone, Risperidone Beats Quetiapine and Quetiapine Beats Olanzapine: An Exploratory Analysis of Head-to-head Comparison Studies of Second-Generation Antipsychotics. *Am J Psychiatry*, 163, 185–194.

42. Every-Palmer S, Howick J (2014). How Evidence-Based Medicine is Failing Due to Biased Trials and Selective Publication. *J Eval Clin Pract*, 20, 908–914.

43. Fleming A (1980). On the Antibacterial Action of Cultures of a Penicillium, with Special Reference to their Use in the Isolation of B.Influenzae. *Rev Infect Dis*, 2, 129–139. (Reprinted from the *Br J Exp Pathol*, 10, 226–236).

44. Sjoding MW, Iwashyna TJ, Dimick JB, Cooke CR (2015). Gaming Hospital-level Pneumonia 30-day Mortality and Readmission Measures by Legitimate Changes to Diagnostic Coding. *Crit Care Med*, 43, 989–995.

45. McNutt R, Hadler MH (2013). How Clinical Guidelines Can Fail Both Doctors and Patients. Scientific American. Avalilable at: http://blogs.scientificamerican.com/guest-blog/2013/11/22/how-clinical-guidelines-can-fail-both-doctors-and-patients/ (Accessed on 30/4/2015).

46. Independent Inquiry into Care Provided by Mid Staffordshire NHS Foundation Trust January 2005–March 2009. Chaired by Robert Francis QC. Available at: https://www.gov.uk/government/publications/independent-inquiry-into-care-provided-by-mid-staffordshire-nhs-foundation-trust-january-2001-to-march-2009 (Accessed on 30/4/2015).

47. Moynihan R, Doust J, Henry D (2012). Preventing Overdiagnosis: How to Stop Harming the Healthy. *BMJ*, 344, 19–23.

48. Swinglehurst D, Greenhalgh T, Roberts C (2012). Computer Templates in Chronic Disease Management: Ethnographic Case Study in General Practice. *BMJ*, 2, e001754.

49. Greenhalgh T (2012). Why do We Always End Up Here? Evidence-Based Medicine's Conceptual cul-de-sacs and Some Off-road Alternative Routes. *J Prim Health Care*, 4, 92–97.

Chapter 8

Evidence-Based Medicine and Medical Professionalism

"Professional competence is the habitual and judicious use of communication, knowledge, technical skills, clinical reasoning, emotions, values, and reflection in daily practice for the benefit of the individual and community being served."

Epstein and Hundert, 2002[1]

"Medical professionalism signifies a set of values, behaviours, and relationships that underpins the trust the public has in doctors. In their day-to-day practice, doctors are committed to: integrity, compassion, altruism, continuous improvement, excellence and working in partnership"

Royal College of Physicians London, 2005[2]

"Professionalism is the basis of medicine's contract with society. Essential to this contract is public trust in physicians, which depends on the integrity of both individual physicians and the whole profession."

Medical Professionalism in the New Millennium:
A Physician Charter 2002[3]

Medical professionalism has received unprecedented attention in recent years reflecting an extraordinary rate of change in the ways health care is delivered and the new challenges facing medicine. Medical science and technology advanced rapidly during the 20th century offering a multitude of new diagnostic and therapeutic opportunities. This also led to increased costs and demand and the need to deliver medical care in more efficient ways. Reforms seeking to achieve this brought new fields of expertise into health care, for example, in management, health economics, policy and advocacy. In addition, changes in social attitudes towards authority meant that the paternalism which was often the basis of doctor–patient relationships in the past became unacceptable and widely publicised medical failures served to remind readers of the fallibility of doctors. As a result, the social context of medicine changed and so did the environment in which it is practiced. Doctors are now caring for patients who are likely to be much better informed about their conditions. In addition, they are working with and often managed by colleagues who may have little or no expertise in clinical medicine and so the environment in which medicine is practiced has changed.

Serious failures in medical ethics and regulation which came to light in the late 20th century reinforced pressure for reforms. The Tuskegee study of the natural history of syphilis in the US between 1932 and 1972 concealed from its participants what the study was about. It withheld treatment with penicillin long after it was known to cure syphilis, and actively sought to block access to treatment from other sources. When the scandal became public in 1972, the US government set up a National Commission for the Protection of Human Subjects in Biomedical and Behavioral Research which published the Belmont report in 1979.[4] In the UK, GP Harold Shipman was convicted of murdering 15 of his patients in 2000; however, a subsequent police investigation indicated that he may have killed as many as 218. The subsequent Shipman Enquiry made several far reaching recommendations, in particular the need to reform the General Medical Council (GMC), which regulates doctors and oversees the maintenance of professional standards in the UK.[5] The results of an enquiry published in 2001[6] into an unusually high number of perioperative deaths at the Bristol paediatric cardiac surgical unit between 1984 and 1995 identified a range of serious failures in the health service due to lack of funding, poor organisation and leadership and inadequate facilities. The report made wide ranging recommendations for improving (i) the care children receive, (ii) the culture in which the service operates, (iii) management and leadership and (iv) life-time competency of professionals. Evidence taken at the Bristol Inquiry also revealed that when hearts were removed during post-mortem examinations, they were frequently retained for later research purposes but without the knowledge or consent of parents or relatives. This led to yet another enquiry into the retention of human tissues at the Royal Liverpool Children's Hospital,[7] where the largest collection of organs was based in the UK. This acknowledged that the research undertaken in this way had contributed to the understanding of complex congenital hearts defects, but also identified the need for reforms which led to the Tissue Act 2004 and creation of the Human Tissue Authority to regulate the handling of human tissues in the UK.

There have of course always been challenges to the concept of professionalism, well exemplified by George Bernard Shaw's much quoted remark, "All professions are a conspiracy against the laity", aimed particularly at the medical profession. Some have argued that medical care has changed and Shaw might take a different view now.[8] However, this seems to me to lend unjustified credence to Shaw's opinions. Despite a remarkable ability to articulate his views, Shaw's judgements on social, political and economic issues were often deeply flawed. For example, he opposed vaccination, which he described as "a filthy piece of witchcraft"; he supported eugenics and he called for the extermination of those in society he regarded as unproductive.[9] The historical basis for Shaw's comment about the medical profession relates to an unequal distribution of power between doctors, patients and the wider society. The knowledge that doctors have or claim to have, it is argued, constructs a social model in which the doctor is dominant. This together with the views expressed by Adam Smith, that the motivation of all trades and professions is self-interest, leads to the notion of an unjust and inefficient society. This continues to be a concern about medical professionalism among many sociologists and economists[10,11] and emanates from two separate arguments. First, that medical professionalism has failed to keep pace with changes in the wider society; this seems less justified now since a lot of change and reform has taken place during the past two decades. The second claims that the power monopoly attributed to the medical profession prohibits the operation of a free market in health care, which could otherwise offer efficiencies and savings. Both of these arguments will continue to be debated with claims on both sides.[12,13] They will undoubtedly continue to drive calls for change in the way medicine is practiced and regulated.

Evidence-Based Medicine (EBM)

The launch of EBM in the 1990s coincided with these events. It promoted new ways to care for patients and in doing so also raised important questions about medical professionalism. Its emphasis on greater accuracy in diagnosis and treatment based on an up to date knowledge of published research, also implied that traditional standards of care were inadequate and needed to be improved. This added to the many other voices arguing that medical professionalism itself should be revisited. However, the concept of a hierarchy of evidence promoted by the EBM movement, which proposed that published literature was of greater value than other forms of evidence in medicine had other wide ranging implications for medical professionalism. Since published research is available for all to access, it follows that doctors and the medical profession no longer hold a unique role in the care of patients. Patients themselves can be much better informed and this changes the relationship between doctor and patient. Others with expertise in aspects of the medical literature might also claim to have a role in the care of patients. In addition the relegation of clinical judgement, in favour of decision making based on published data, which the EBM movement argued for, has profound implications for how patients are cared for.

EBM has therefore had a significant impact on the way doctors work and on medical professionalism (Box 8.1). The EBM movement advocated that doctors should be aware of the best research and to implement it in caring for patients. They should know when treatments and diagnostic methods are superseded by more effective or safer ones and use them in line with guidelines. They should aim to reduce the potential risks and harms that accompany many diagnostic tests and treatments. Ineffective treatments should not

---

Box 8.1   Doctors Practicing EBM should:

1. Achieve greater accuracy in diagnosis and treatment;
2. Minimise harm;
3. Remain up to date with published research;
4. Be aware of guidelines;
5. Avoid ineffective therapies;
6. Reduce waste.

be used and waste avoided. None of these of course are new standards which doctors have been required to meet. Nevertheless, they frame the obligations on doctors in a new way. EBM was advocated as a new paradigm of medical practice based on the claim that many aspects of medical practice were inadequate and needed to be improved. It followed from this that medical professionalism itself needed to be revised. And so EBM in effect became another voice calling for an overhaul of medical professionalism.

As the 20th century closed, these voices reached a climax and could not be left unanswered. In the US there was deep frustration over rising and uncontrolled health care costs, claims of greed against corporate health providers and drug companies against a backdrop of unsustainable and unaffordable costs for many citizens.[14] It was claimed that the public no longer had trust in medical professionalism and the rise of the citizen's right to choose as a customer made the current concept of medical professionalism obsolete.[14] Within the medical profession itself feelings of disquiet and frustration were also growing amid fears that the changes in healthcare delivery systems were threatening the values implicit in medical professionalism.[3] In the UK, medical professionalism was debated against a backdrop of the Shipman murders and the Bristol enquiry and also within the context of unprecedented reforms in the way health care is managed and delivered as discussed in Chapter 4. Contributions to the discussion therefore were advanced from different perspectives on healthcare.

Health Policy and Management

Groups interested in health policy and health management, notably the King's Fund,[15,16] The Nuffield Trust, The Health Foundation[17] (formerly the Private Patients Plan Trust and now the largest UK health policy charity), The Institute for Public Policy Research[18] and the Department of Health[19] published in-house documents reinforcing the need for changes in medical professionalism citing all of the challenges mentioned above. These tended to be particularly concerned that medical professionalism should embrace cooperative, productive and respectful interaction among doctors and the increasing number of stake-holders involved in healthcare. A new compact between doctors and society was advocated in which clinicians played a greater role in management and leadership in health care and engaged in improving health services.[15,16] Others stressed the changing age structure, ethnicity and gender of health workers. In addition, the levels of expertise among nurses, physiotherapists and other carers needed to be reflected in a new commitment to teamwork in medical professionalism.[18] Although some expressed a much greater opposition to the concept of professionalism as a social construct[19] there was also fairly unanimous agreement that doctors remained one of the most trusted groups in society.

The Royal College of Physicians (RCP)

As in almost every other country in the western world, doctors in the UK were also concerned by the new challenges they faced and the direction professionalism was heading. In 2004, the RCP set up a working party to consider the role of doctors in society and the meaning, purpose, relevance and future of medical professionalism. Its report[20] (Box 8.2) published in 2005 was broadly welcomed.[21] It recognised that public trust in medicine had been undermined by serious well publicised failures, that expectations of the public and of politicians had changed radically over the past half century, and also that some political and managerial changes in health care had jeopardised the quality of patient care and the ability of doctors to meet their professional obligations. In doing so, it acknowledged that there was an urgent need to reconsider and redefine medical professionalism.

In its recommendations, the report confirmed the working party's view that medical professionalism was an essential element of medicine which underpins public trust in doctors. At its heart is the relationship between patients and doctors in which doctors must be committed to:

(i)   *Integrity,*
(ii) *Compassion,*
(iii) *Altruism,*
(iv) *Continuous improvement,*
(v)   *Excellence,*
(vi) *Working in partneship.*

In redefining professionalism, the report argued that some traditional notions should be abandoned. The term *mastery,* which could mean a skilful

Box 8.2   Medical Professionalism.

Essential Elements

1. Integrity
2. Compassion
3. Altruism
4. Continuous improvement
5. Excellence
6. Working in partnership
7. Appropriate accountability

Concepts Modified

1. Excellence rather than competence
2. Judgement rather than art
3. Moral contract rather than social contract

Concepts Abandoned

1. Mastery
2. Autonomy
3. Privilege

use of knowledge, could also suggest control, power and authority which have no place in medicine. *Autonomy* was liable to *misinterpretion*. Doctors should be able to advise patients in their best interests free from external interference. However, autonomy could also be understood to mean a right to self-regulate, or clinical autonomy could be taken to mean a right to act independently of medical evidence; neither of which is acceptable. *Privilege* too in the sense of immunity from liability was also considered inappropriate.

The report also considered three concepts which should be altered to reflect modern views. *Competence* should be replaced by *excellence* to indicate that just having an ability to practice medicine is insufficient, and that it needs to be to an eminent or meritorious level. Despite its long use, the word *art* applied to medicine was felt to be too non-specific and general and should be replaced by *judgement* meaning the application of reasoning in conjunction with relevant evidence to solve or mitigate clinical problems. The relationship between doctors and society is sometime referred to as a *social contract*, which the working party believed did not adequately reflect the importance of integrity and honesty in medical professionalism and suggested *moral contract* as better substitute. The working party felt there were strong grounds for retaining notions of *knowledge, skills, science, profession, society, service, commitment and integrity.* However, the idea of medicine as a vocation was controversial; many believe it is a job like any other. There was also concern that the idea of *vocation* could imply an element of divine calling and resonances of doctors as "God-like" in status. On the other hand, the college was keen to foster a sense of passion and ethical commitment about a career in medicine.

There was unanimity that doctors should be *accountable.* The working party stressed the value of *appropriate accountability,* meaning that it should be to enable doctors to work in the best interests of their patients without the fear of unfair penalty for errors made unintentionally and in good faith. There was concern that an unthinking accountability in a context of unbalanced media stories of medical scares could lead to an atmosphere of suspicion that doctors in general were not acting in the best interests of their patients. The report also expressed concern that excessive managerial control often erodes trust by implying the subject controlled cannot otherwise be relied on.[22] The concept of *altruism* as an element of medical professionalism caused most dissent. While altruism meaning having regard for others and unselfishness are uncontroversial, it could also be construed as meaning that doctors should sacrifice their own lives or the well-being of their families for their profession or that doctors are somehow morally better than others, both of which are unacceptable. The report was particularly concerned to emphasise the central role of *the patient, partnership, well being and human dignity* in medical professionalism. These three elements are central to medical professionalism but also encompass its most complex and interacting responsibilities. On the one hand, doctors must place the patient at the centre of their work, but at the same time cannot set this as a reason to exclude themselves from accepted practice standards such as EBM or cooperating with healthcare management and resource allocation. The report set out its view that the corollary to this was also necessary; that health care needed to be managed in a way that enables doctors to fulfill their professional obligations. It also acknowledged doctors' concerns that health service reforms were often an impediment to delivering the best care for those most in need and that at its best professionalism meant challenging political power to ensure that health service delivery is based on reliable evidence. The future of medical professionalism would depend on maintaining a culture that fostered the values which underpin it at all levels in the service.

General Medical Council

GMC regulates doctors in the UK. All doctors must be registered with it and it has the power to investigate and reprimand doctors and to restrict or suspend their right to practice. It therefore has a particular role in relation to medical professionalism. It provides guidance to doctors and sets out standards they must meet. In previous guidance notes, the GMC had not referred to the duties of doctors in terms of medical professionalism and its absence was noted by the RCP's working party (p. 23),[17] with a suggestion that it would be helpful to do so. In its recent guidance (Box 8.3), the GMC seems to have taken this on board, referring to "good doctors" and "professionalism in action". Overall GMC guidance on the duties of doctors is closely aligned with the views of the RCP working party, but the GMC sets the patient as a more central priority than the RCP report. GMC guidance is presented in four themes.

The GMC is quite specific in stating that, patients must be the first concern of doctors and that they must provide a good standard of care by keeping up to date. They must take action promptly should they become aware of risks to the safety and dignity of patients', including those cared for by their colleagues. Patients must be treated as individuals, with respect and as partners in making decisions about their health. Doctors must be aware of and respond to patients' preferences and also respect their rights to privacy and confidentiality. Doctors must also work in partnership with colleagues to best serve the interests of patients. Patients must be able to trust their doctors with their lives and health. Therefore, maintaining trust is a key obligation of doctors. They must be honest and open and act with integrity, treat patients and colleagues fairly and never abuse patients' or the public's trust in the profession.

Box 8.3   GMC Guidance on the Duties of Doctors.

Knowledge Skill and Performance

1. Care of patients must be the first concern.
2. Doctors must provide a good standard of care by:
   o Keeping professional knowledge and skill up to date.
   o Knowing their limits and working within them.

Safety and Quality

1. Act promptly to protect patient safety, dignity and comfort.
2. Protect and promote the health of patients and the public.

Communication, Partnership and Teamwork

1. Treat patients as individuals and respect their dignity
   o Treat patients politely and considerately.
   o Respect patients right to confidentiality.
2. Work in partnership with patients
   o Listen to, and respond to, their concerns and preferences.
   o Provide the information they want or need in a way they can understand.
   o Respect patients' right to reach decisions with you about their treatment and care.
   o Support patients own efforts to improve and maintain their health.
3. Work with colleagues in ways that best serve patients' interests.

Maintaining Trust

1. Be honest and open and act with integrity.
2. Never discriminate unfairly against patients or colleagues.
3. Never abuse your patients' trust in you or the public's trust in the profession.

Doctors are personally accountable for their professional practice and must always be prepared to justify their decisions and actions.

Professionalism in Practice

These concepts of medical professionalism discard older ideas which are no longer acceptable. There is an explicit attempt to exclude anything which might lend support to old charges of doctors being God-like, paternalistic, or socially or morally superior. Rather doctors are seen as having acquired knowledge and skill which can be of service to others and that service must be done in accordance with the regulatory guidelines. This in practice is recognised by organisations which support doctors in the event of errors and mistakes,[23] in the training of medical students[24] and more widely in medicine.[21]

EBM and Medical Professionalism

The working party of the RCP went to some length to recognise EBM as an important element of medical professionalism. Its report clarified that (i) doctors must base their practice on reliable evidence, (ii) that there is no overriding autonomy to excuse not doing so and (iii) doctors must be prepared to explain their actions in terms of reasoned application of evidence to solve or ameliorate patients' problems. The report therefore leaves no doubt (if it were not already self-evident) that EBM is an integral part of medical professionalism. However, it is equally explicit that medical professionalism concerns much more than the application of the latest research evidence; it goes far beyond what the EBM movement claimed to be a new paradigm for practicing medicine and is in conflict with several tenets of its advocacy.

Evidence and Judgement

In its efforts to promote the application of research evidence to medical practice, the EBM movement de-emphasised the value of reasoning based on the understanding of pathophysiological mechanisms, clinical experience and acquired knowledge as the sole basis for making clinical decisions. Instead a new paradigm of medical practice was advocated which prioritised an up to date knowledge of published research. This led to the notion of a hierarchy of evidence in which comparative research was more valuable than clinical judgement.[25,26] This has been disputed as discussed in Chapter 5. It also raises potential concerns in relation to medical professionalism. However, much of this can be traced to differences in what is understood by "clinical judgement" and how the term is used. In its advocacy of published research, the EBM movement argued that a systematic analysis of it is more reliable than an intuitive guess, referred to as "expert clinical judgement", based on accumulated knowledge.[26] In reality, I suspect that few would disagree with this. However, this is not the meaning of the term "clinical judgement" as it is understood in relation to clinical medicine or medical professionalism. Forming a judgement about an area of research is not a clinical matter and is not specific to clinical medicine or to clinicians. It is simply a judgement. For clinicians and in the context of medical professionalism, clinical judgement refers to decisions made in a clinical context in relation to an individual patient; it is "the application of critical reasoning to a problem presented by a patient in order to arrive at an opinion about how to solve or ameliorate that problem"[20] based on the most reliable evidence and taking into account the patient's wishes. The use of evidence as advocated by EBM is an integral part of making clinical judgements, but it is just one aspect of it. It would not be acceptable for example to ignore particular aspects of an individual patient's needs or wishes on the basis of some published research. Neither would it be acceptable to ignore the most reliable evidence on the basis of some personal belief of opinion. Thus, clinical judgements are at the heart of medical practice and medical professionalism; they must include reliable evidence in their deliberations, but they cannot be relegated in favour of or replaced by the application of any single source of evidence.

Guidelines, Rules and Clinical Judgement

Clinical guidelines provide a valuable source of information for medical practice. As discussed in Chapter 7, they are based on a synthesis of research related to the management of particular illnesses. They are also the most important practical expression of EBM. Their wide acceptance and the high regard in which they are held is an indication that EBM itself is now accepted as the norm in medicine. Medical professionalism requires that doctors must be aware of guidelines relevant to their practice and be committed to keeping themselves up to date on them. However, guidelines too are just one element of clinical practice; they cannot be used to excuse disregarding the wishes and needs of an individual patient. Medical professionalism requires that guidelines are considered and applied where appropriate in making clinical decisions. A reasoned decision not to adhere to them can be made in individual cases, but in doing so doctors must be prepared to explain why.

Rule-following in medicine has also been suggested to be superior to clinical judgement.[26] But here again the term clinical judgement is misused. The argument usually arises in relation to the systematic use of criteria in making a diagnosis. When the symptoms and signs of a condition vary considerably between patients, noting the presence or absence of particular features and knowledge of their significance can improve diagnostic accuracy. As discussed in Chapter 5, this is well known in clinical medicine and has been taught to medical students for many decades.[27] Whether or not a clinical diagnosis is made with the use of such criteria does not alter the fact that it remains a clinical diagnosis. Diagnostic criteria are elicited using clinical skills and the diagnosis remains a clinical one, which will contribute to a clinical judgement in managing the patient. It does not follow that because the use of diagnostic criteria can improve clinical diagnoses they can somehow replace either clinical skills or clinical judgements. By the same token, rule-following would not be an acceptable reason for failing to make clinical judgements based on individual patients' needs.

Medical Professionalism in the Health Service

Appropriate accountability is an essential part of medical professionalism. To enable this, doctors are required to maintain their commitment to professional values throughout their careers. This is achieved by an annual appraisal and revalidation every five years. The former consists of a yearly review of their professional work based on collected evidence and is centred on the clinical interaction with patients. Revalidation is required to maintain a licence to practice medicine and is done by the GMC every five years based on satisfactory submissions of annual appraisals.[28] Both appraisal and revalidation are essentially concerned with ensuring that every doctor continues to meet the standards of medical professionalism. Misconceptions about the roles of clinical judgement, guidelines and rule-following which arose from the EBM movements efforts to prioritise published research may have contributed to confusion about medical professionalism and the purpose of appraisal and revalidation. The notion that clinical judgement can be replaced by guidelines and rule-following would, if accepted, reduce clinical medicine to a technical activity in which medical professionalism was redundant. This in turn may have been behind an idea within the Department of Health that appraisal of doctors was about clinical performance rather than professional development. Views expressed in one of its early publications that "Appraisal should include data on clinical performance, training and education, audit, concerns raised and serious clinical complaints, application of relevant clinical guidelines, relationships with patients and colleagues, teaching and research activities, and personal and organisational effectiveness" clearly worried the RCP's Working Party which went to some lengths to correct it (p. 36).[20] Much of that confusion has now resolved and accountability of doctors is accepted as the responsibility of the GMC based on appraisal and revalidation.

Clinical and Non-Clinical Professionalism and the Role of EBM

Most but not all doctors work with patients and for them professionalism is centred on their clinical practice. There are, however, many other crucial roles for doctors in medicine, for example in public health and epidemiology. Their duties and responsibilities are to protect the health of the wider community, mainly by promoting prevention measures and managing illnesses, which arise and spread in populations such as epidemics. Research at a community level also provides powerful insights into the state of health not only in nations but also globally. It is important for example to understand the geographical, ethnic and social distribution of ill health in order to better deliver prevention and care. Research at a population level can also reveal important information about how health services deliver care. For example, the challenge of over-diagnosis discussed in Chapter 7 was uncovered by epidemiological research studying survival in large numbers of people. It is clear then that research derived from population studies can have important bearing to the way individual patients are cared for. In the same way the effectiveness of prevention measures at a population level has a major impact on health service needs. For example, we now have a growing and alarming rise in over-weight and obesity in most western populations, which is the most important cause of rising levels of type II diabetes. In England, the cost of caring for patients with diabetes has now risen to almost 10% of the entire budget for GP practices.[29] It is inevitable and appropriate therefore that knowledge in all areas of medicine should be used to help improve health at all levels.

The impetus for EBM also arose from epidemiological research suggesting that many aspects of health service delivery lacked a strong evidence base resulting in suboptimal or ineffective treatments and waste. The main concern which EBM sought to correct was that clinicians were relying too much on their knowledge of the literature and not enough on up to date systematic appraisal of it. And the solutions developed have largely been derived from epidemiological methods, such as systematic reviews and the Cochrane Collaboration. These have served medicine well. However, they have also contributed to an unbalanced rhetoric about the challenges facing medicine. Both the criticisms and advocacy of EBM have focused almost exclusively on clinical medicine and even then have been largely restricted to the treatment of individual patients. In contrast, large areas of medicine and health care in serious need of an evidence base such as the management of public health and the health service are ignored. Clinical medicine has benefited from the reforms this has stimulated. However, it may also have been harmed by some EBM rhetoric. The EBM movement's criticism was exclusively directed at clinical medicine and some of it was misjudged including the notion that clinical judgement might be replaced by rule-following and guidelines.[30] This I suggest partly explains evidence gathered by the RCP from many clinicians who believed that their professionalism was being eroded and that clinical medicine risked becoming a technical box ticking activity.[20] It is noteworthy too that about this time clinicians were removed from senior management roles in healthcare and replaced by managers from industry or non-clinical specialties.

Medical Professionalism and Leadership

There is now unanimity that better leadership is needed to improve the quality of care in health services[31] and the lack of clinicians engaged in leadership roles is seen as a serious problem.[32] This has its origins in reforms of health service organisation at the end of the 20th century which replaced the old cog-wheel system, run largely by clinicians, by one based on private sector experience, which hired non-medical managers instead of senior clinicians.[33]

Although initially this seemed a deliberate policy to change the culture of the service, it also became clear that few clinicians were willing to engage with it.[34,35] The management culture of the NHS changed rapidly, but progress in improving the efficiency of the service was poor and this was soon blamed on a lack of clinicians involved in management.[36] Poor leadership continues to be a challenge for the NHS[31] and failure to engage clinicians in it is recognised by some as a contributing error.[37] Reports on the problem appear at regular intervals.[32,38] After two decades of reforms, as recently as 2013 many clinicians remain sceptical of health service management and tensions between clinicians and managers persist,[32] despite clear evidence that this has been a major contributing factor in recent major failings as at Mid Staffordshire.[39] Various remedies have been proposed to improve clinicians' engagement in NHS management over the years. Interviews with current and former health managers themselves point to the high risks in taking on senior roles with the average tenure for CEOs being 700 days, a culture of scapegoating individuals, and impossible challenges to "fix the unfixable".[40] One consultant who took up a role as CEO and had to resign due to problems that were longstanding and beyond his control added to these, the risk that doctors might be placed in a conflicted position, having to compromise their values to meet some short term objectives in a managerial culture where blame is common.[41] Perhaps the scale of the problems revealed at Mid Staffordshire by the Francis enquiry will force a long needed change in culture. At least it is now formally recognised that patients' experiences must be at the centre of the service delivery and recent guidelines published by the National Institute for Clinical Excellence (NICE) add weight to this.[42] That report and reactions to it seem to illustrate why the problem has been so intractable but also how it can be solved.

In its guidance, NICE uses the word "professional" 23 times over 29 pages,[42] and in doing so refers to the professional work of doctors and nurses in caring for patients as the basis on which a patient centred service must be implemented, thus recognising the nature, significance and role of medical professionalism. In contrast, it is virtually absent in the rhetoric of experts who teach and research NHS management. Thus, for example, in a document of 206 pages on medical leadership in the NHS funded by the National Institute for Health Research,[32] the word professional appears 102 times, but nowhere does it actually refer to the professional roles of doctors and nurses. It discusses "professional organisations" and "professional bureaucracies". In a historical section, it refers to "older professional values" but never discusses what it considers to be newer professional values. It refers to "professional autonomy" meaning autonomous in terms of managerial control, but not as a concept understood (and abandoned[20]) in terms of medical professionalism. It refers to "tensions between professional values and organisational values" but nowhere does it explore what these might be or why they have arisen. This seems to me to be emblematic of and the primary reason for the recurring failure of in NHS management, namely, the failure adequately to understand and acknowledge medical professionalism. The notion that patients' experience of the health service can be improved simply by measuring it more often[43] fails to grasp this and is unconvincing.[44] This lack of coherence between health service managers and clinicians is freely admitted by managers themselves as one director expressed it "We haven't got clinicians who have swallowed the gospel according to the Trust. You don't get that with clinicians. Sometime people ask: Why aren't the doctors more corporate? Doctors just won't put the Trust at the top of their hierarchy of values. They just won't do it". Here the speaker understands that the root of the problem is perceived conflicts between management imperatives and the professional obligations of clinicians, but appears to have no idea of what lies behind this tension or how it has arisen. The consequences of this misalignment are perfectly illustrated in an independent enquiry into an attempt to transfer dermatological services to a private company in Nottingham.[45] The report concluded that the "unmitigated disaster" which resulted was principally due to a lack of understanding and failure to acknowledge the professional values of the clinicians concerned.

This is perhaps not surprising considering the recent NHS history. The introduction of administrative reforms in the NHS during the 1990s took place against a backdrop of perceived failures in medical professionalism and its regulation. Enquiries into the murders carried out by GP Harold Shipman[5] and failings in paediatric surgery at Bristol[6] and other failings in the health service[7] undermined confidence in regulation of doctors and in the profession generally. Despite the fact that these scandals identified widespread failings it seemed to be failed medical professionalism which was mainly held[46] to be accountable and needed to be reformed. At this time too, the day to day professional role of doctors was being questioned by the rhetoric of EBM which suggested that the clinical judgements doctors make every day are unreliable and could be replaced by guidelines and rule-following as discussed in Chapter 5. The view that professionalism in general is really about self-interest and empire building was also common.[19] Added to this, there were criticisms that medical leadership was too paternalistic based on hierarchies that were too steep and needed to be more distributive;[47] ironic, since at this point clinical leadership was relatively absent from the NHS. Airline pilots were given as an example for clinicians to follow with their flatter hierarchy of cockpit management;[48] although this suggestion has receded following evidence that one of the worst flight disasters in recent history was shown to have resulted precisely from a lack of leadership based on knowledge and experience.[49]

Faced with the major challenge of overhauling, the health service in the context of almost constant change, new managers from industry, with little experience of healthcare, would not have regarded understanding medical professionalism as their priority. This seems hardly to have changed; the deliberations of non-medical managers continue to show little evidence of awareness of the professional obligations of nurses and doctors, or acknowledgement of the need for a service environment in which they can flourish[32,43,50] despite the fact that NICE guidance pinpoints both as central to putting patients at the centre of the service.[42] This I suggest is the primary reason for clinicians avoiding direct involvement in NHS service management. After almost two decades of health service reform including the medical regulation of clinicians, the GMC has made it clear that their relations with and behaviour towards patients remain central to medical professionalism and doctors licence to practice.[28] It is difficult to envisage clinicians being willing participants in management systems which they perceive do not understand, acknowledge or respect this. It seems extraordinary that this continues to hold back progress in the NHS,[32] given that caring for patients is the common objective of all who work in it and there are no clear solutions in view. But perhaps there is a hidden logic to this. Fundamentally, the long term direction of the NHS remains unclear. Despite almost continuous reforms over the past three decades, as discussed in Chapter 4, the current rhetoric at the highest levels remains "transformative change is needed" and "the NHS has to change" without any clear idea of what this might lead to. Given this, it may be more desirable to have a cadre of senior managers who are less hamstrung by the GMC, but can be fired at will if things go wrong. In this context, the GMC is clear that doctors undertaking management roles which can be done by non-medical staff are still subject to its regulations and they can be punished for decisions which adversely affect patients including those with whom they have had no direct contact. It seems likely therefore that unless and until medical professionalism is acknowledged and recognised at a senior levels within the health service it will continue to act as a barrier to clinicians engaging in management roles. EBM could play an important role in reversing this. Health service reforms have come and gone over the past two decades in a vacuum of evidence about their effects and for this to have occurred in the era of EBM must surely be an historic irony. A campaign for evidence-based Health Service Management is desperately needed and the advocacy and rhetorical skills of the EBM movement place it in an ideal position to do this. It would also give clinicians more confidence that their involvement in service management could be evidence-based, less prone to short term political manipulation, and their actions more readily justified on the basis of available evidence.

Conclusions

Medical professionalism has received unprecedented attention in many countries during the past two decades, prompted by sharp increases in demand for health services and rising costs. In the UK, well-publicised cases of medical failures and subsequent public enquiries called for an overhaul of medical regulation. The launch of the EBM movement coincided with these events and its criticisms of clinical medicine in not being sufficiently evidence-based added to those calling for change. Health policy and management think tanks waded in arguing that medical professionalism vested too much power in doctors, needed to be more responsive and cooperative towards other stakeholders in the health service and to be more responsive to management and availability of resources.

In response to this medical leaders in several western countries published a physician's charter for the new millennium in 2002. In the UK, the Royal College of Physicians, London set up a working party to consider and redefine medical professionalism which reported in 2005. This set out in detail the basis on which it saw medical professionalism for the future; it emphasised integrity, compassion, altruism, continuous improvement, excellence, working in partnership and accountability, as central to maintaining trust. Subsequently the GMC, which regulates doctors in the UK, updated its guidance, most recently in 2013. This is broadly in line with the RCP's report, but more explicitly puts the care of patients as the primary concern for doctors.

EBM therefore has had an important impact in highlighting the need for reform of clinical medicine. It has also been important in ensuring that clinical practice is not only based on reliable evidence, but that this is recognised as a professional value doctors must hold. However, some aspects of the rhetoric of EBM movement, especially in its early days were contrary to accepted tenets of medical professionalism. Its notion of a hierarchy of evidence with published research trumping clinical judgement was wrong. So too was its advocacy of rule-following as a substitute for clinical judgement. Some of this can be attributed to a misunderstanding of the term clinical judgement by members of the movement unfamiliar with clinical medicine. Nevertheless it contributed to a sense that clinicians and medical professionalism were flawed.

As the integrity and reliability of medical professionalism was being questioned, senior clinical leaders were replaced by non-clinical managers in health service roles, initially by design, but in time it became clear that clinicians were avoiding them. This has continued and is now seen as a serious block to progress in the NHS. This can be attributed in part to lingering out dated attitudes towards medicine some of which were the result of the rhetoric of the EBM movement's advocacy. The most important impediments reflect tensions between the values which clinicians must uphold and the failure to acknowledge and respect these within the culture of health service management. Recent guidance from the GMC has reinforced those values and NICE has added to this by placing the experience, dignity and wellbeing of patients at the forefront of what the health service does. Neither of these will be fully realised until medical professionalism is adequately recognised and encouraged in the health service.

The EBM movement has potentially an important role in this. Its most important step would be to direct its celebrated rhetorical skills and advocacy to campaign for transparency in health service management and pressing for an end to the vacuum of evidence surrounding recent and proposed service reforms. This would encourage clinicians to believe that their involvement in management could be based on evidence rather than diktat and that the professional values they must uphold would not be conflicted for short term imperatives.

References

1. Epstein RM, Hundert EM (2002). Defining and Assessing Professional Competence. *JAMA*, 287(2), 226–235.
2. Doctors in Society (2005). Medical Professionalism in a Changing World. Report of a Working Party, Royal College of Physicians London. Available at: https://www.rcplondon.ac.uk/sites/default/files/documents/doctors_in_society_reportweb.pdf (Accessed on 11/5/2015).
3. Medical Professionalism in the New Millennium (2002). A Physician Charter; Project of the ABIM Foundation, ACP–ASIM Foundation, and European Federation of Internal Medicine. *Ann Intern Med*, 136, 243–246.
4. The Belmont Report; Ethical Principles and Guidelines for the protection of human subjects of research. Available at: http://archive.hhs.gov/ohrp/human subjects/guidance/belmont.htm (Accessed on 13/5/2015).
5. The Shipman Inquiry, Sixth report (2005). Shipman: the Final Report. Available at: http://webarchive.nationalarchives.gov.uk/20090808154959/http://www. the-shipman-inquiry.org.uk/finalreport.asp (Accessed on 11/12/2015).
6. The Bristol Royal Infirmary Enquiry (2001). The Report of the Public Inquiry into Children's Heart Surgery at the Bristol Royal Infirmary 1984–1995: Learning from Bristol. Available at: http://webarchive.nationalarchives.gov. uk/20090811143745/http:/www.bristol-inquiry.org.uk/final_report/the_ report.pdf (Accessed on 11/12/2015).
7. The Royal Liverpool Children's Inquiry (2001). The Royal Liverpool Children's Inquiry Report. Available at: http://webarchive.nationalarchives.gov.uk/20060 715141954/rlcinquiry.org.uk (Accessed on 11/12/2015).
8. Donaldson L (2003). Commentary: The Doctor's Dilemma: a response. *Inte J Epidemiol*, 32, 916–917.
9. Shaw GB (1934). The Listener London, February 7, 1934.
10. Friedson E (1970). *Profession of Medicine: a Study of the Sociology of Applied Knowledge.* Chicago: University of Chicago Press.
11. Salvage J (2002). Rethinking Professionalism: The First Step for Patient Focused Care?. Future Health Worker Project, Available at: http://www.ippr.org/assets/

media/uploadedFiles/projects/Rethinking%20Professionalism%20PDF?
noredirect=1. (Accessed on 14/5/2015).

12. Roy A (2012). The Myth of 'Free-Market' American Health Care — And The
Reality of Singapore's. Forbes Magazine 3/9/2012. Available at: http://www.
forbes.com/sites/theapothecary/2012/03/09/the-myth-of-free-market-ameri-
can-health-care/ (Accessed on 15/5/2015).

13. Kantarjian H, Zwelling L (2013). Cancer Drug Prices and the Free-Market
Forces. *Cancer*, 119, 3903–3905.

14. Berwick DM (2009). The Epitaph of Profession. *Br J Gen Pract*, 59, 128–131.

15. Rosen R, Dewar S (2004). On Being A Doctor: Redefining Medical
Professionalism for Better Patient Care. Kings Fund. Available at: http://www.
kingsfund.org.uk/sites/files/kf/field/field_publication_file/on-being-a-doctor-
redefining-medical-professionalism-better-patient-care-rebecca-rosen-steve-
dewar-kings-fund-1-november-2004.pdf (Accessed on 14/5/2015).

16. Levenson R, Dewar R, Shepherd S (2008). Understanding Doctors: Harnessing
Professionalism. King's Fund. Available at: http://www.kingsfund.org.uk/sites/files/
kf/Understanding-Doctors-Harnessing-professionalism-Ros-Levenson-Steve-
Dewar-Susan-Shepherd-Kings-Fund-May-2008_0.pdf (Accessed on 15/5/2015).

17. Christmas S, Millward L (2011). New Medical Professionalism: A scoping
Report for the Health Foundation. Available at: http://www.health.org.uk/pub-
lic/cms/75/76/313/2733/New%20medical%20professionalism.pdf?realName=
JOGEKF.pdf (Accessed on 15/5/2015).

18. Salvage J (2002). Rethinking Professionalism: The First Step for Patient Focused
Care?. Institute for Public Policy Research. Available at: http://www.ippr.org/
assets/media/uploadedFiles/projects/Rethinking%20Professionalism%20.
PDF?noredirect=1 (Accessed on 15/5/2015).

19. Clayton H (2005). Submission to Doctors in Society, Royal College of
Physicians, London. Available at: https://www.rcplondon.ac.uk/sites/default/
files/documents/docs_in_socs_tech_navigable.pdf (Accessed on 15/5/2015).

20. Doctors in Society Medical Professionalism in a Changing World (2005). Report
of a Working Party, Royal College of Physicians. Available at: https://www.rcplon-
don.ac.uk/sites/default/files/documents/doctors_in_society_reportweb.pdf
(Accessed on 15/5/2015).

21. Horton R (2005). Medicine: the Prosperity of Virtue. *Lancet*, 366, 1985–1987
and 2006 367, 646–648.

22. O'Neill O (2004). Accountability, Trust, and Informed Consent in Medical
Practice and Research. *Clin Med*, 4, 269–276.

23. Professionalism — An MPS Guide. Medical Protection Society, 2013. Available
at: http://www.medicalprotection.org/docs/default-source/pdfs/Booklet-PDFs/
professionalism-an-mps-guide.pdf?sfvrsn=2 (Accesed on 17/5/2015).

24. Professionalism. Southampton University, Medical Education Development Unit. Available at: http://www.southampton.ac.uk/medu/curriculum_design_and_delivery/professionalism.page (Accessed on 17/5/2015).

25. The Evidence based Medicine Working Group (1992). The Evidence Based Medicine: A New Approach to Teaching and Practice of Medicine. *JAMA*, 268, 2420–2425.

26. Howick J. *The philosophy of Evidence-Based Medicine*. Wiley Blackwell BMJ Books 2011. Oxford: Blackwell-Wiley.

27. Duckett Jones T (1944). The Diagnosis of Rheumatic Fever. *JAMA*. 126(8), 481–484.

28. Supporting Information for Appraisal and Revalidation (2012). General Medical Council. Available at: http://www.gmc-uk.org/doctors/revalidation/9612.asp (Accessed on 21/5/2015).

29. Prescribing for Diabetes, England — 2005–2006 to 2013–2014. Health and Social Care Information Centre. Available at: http://www.hscic.gov.uk/catalogue/PUB14681. (Accessed on 21/5/2015).

30. Greenhalgh T, Howick J, Maskrey N (2014). Evidence Based Medicine: A Movement in Crisis? *BMJ*, 348, g3725.

31. Ham C (2014). Strengthening Leadership in the NHS. The Rose and Dalton Reviews are Welcome but there are No Easy Answers. *BMJ*, 348, g1685.

32. Dickinson H, Ham C, Snelling I, Spurgeon P (2013). Are We There Yet? Models of Medical Leadership and their Effectiveness: An Exploratory Study. Available at: http://kingsfund.blogs.com/health_management/2013/04/are-we-there-yet-models-of-medical-leadership-and-their-effectiveness-an-exploratory-study-final-report.html (Accessed on 11/12/2015).

33. Horton R (2002). The Doctor's Role in Advocacy. *The Lancet*, 359, 458.

34. Morrison PE, Heineke J (1992), Why do Health Care Practitioners Resist Quality Management? *Qual Prog*, 25(4), 51–55.

35. Shekelle PG (2002). Why Don't Physicians Enthusiastically Support Quality Improvement Programmes? *Qual Saf Health Care*, 11, 6.

36. Gallop R, Whitby E, Buchanan D et al., (2004). Influencing Sceptical Staff to become Supporters of Service Improvement: A Qualitative study of Doctors'and Managers' views. *Qual Saf Health Care*, 13(2), 108–114.

37. Shapiro J, Rashid S (2011). Leadership in the NHS: Professionals Respond Better to Inclusion than Coercion. *BMJ*, 342, d3375.

38. King's Fund, Future Leadership and Management in the NHS (2011). No More Heroes. Available at: http://www.kingsfund.org.uk/publications/nhs_leadership.html (Accessed on 23/5/2015).

39. Francis R (2013). Report of the Mid-Staffordshire NHS Foundation Trust Public Inquiry. HC 947. Stationery Office.

40. Vize R (2015). Why Would a Consultant Think of Going into Management? *BMJ*, 350, 16–18. *BMJ*, 2015; 350 doi: http://dx.doi.org/10.1136/bmj.h922 (Published 24 February 2015), *BMJ*, 350, h922.

41. Newbold M (2015). Time to Tackle Managerial Culture. *BMJ*, 350, h922.

42. Patient Experience in Adult NHS Services: Improving the Experience of Care for People using Adult NHS Services, 2012. Available at: http://www.nice.org. uk/guidance/cg138 (Accessed on 23/5/2015).

43. Eaton S, Collins A, Coulter A, Elwyn G, Grazin N, Roberts S (2012). Putting Patients First NICE Guidance on the Patient Experience is a Welcome Small Step on a Long Journey. *BMJ*, 344, e2006.

44. Edwards A (2012). Positive Leadership is Key. *BMJ*, 344, e3080.

45. Clough C. Final Report: Independent Review of Nottingham Dermatology Services. Available at: http://bit.ly/1IARWyg (Accessed on 12/7/2015).

46. Smith R (1998). British Medicine will be Transformed by the Bristol case. *BMJ*, 316, 1917.

47. Sexton JB, Thomas EJ, Helmreich RL (2000). Error, Stress and Teamwork in Medicine and Aviation: Cross Sectional Surveys. *BMJ*, 320, 745–749.

48. McCulloch P, Mishra A, Handa A, Dale T, Hirst G, Catchpole K (2009). The Effects of Aviation-Style Non-Technical Skills Training on Technical Performance and Outcome in the Operating Theatre. *Qual Saf Health Care*. 18, 109–115.

49. Bhangu A1, Bhangu S, Stevenson J, Bowley DM (2013). Lessons for Surgeons in the Final Moments of Air France Flight 447. *World J Surg*, 37, 1185–1192.

50. Webster R (2015). It's Time to be Honest About Future NHS Funding. *BMJ*, 350, H1978.

Chapter 9

The Future of Evidence-Based Medicine

Efforts to ensure that the care of patients is based on reliable evidence have a long history in medicine. These earlier efforts may have been overshadowed by the campaigning tactics available in our own times, but the desire for it and awareness of the need for it have not been less in the past. The new campaign for Evidence-Based Medicine (EBM) of the early 1990s was launched at a time when the values of medical professionalism were being re-evaluated and perhaps its most enduring legacy to medicine will be that it contributed to ensuring that EBM is now formally recognised within that value system. There seems little doubt therefore that EBM is here to stay. Despite this, or perhaps because of the extent of the impact of EBM in medicine, it has tended to overwhelm other values in medicine, leading some to call for reform of its position within that value system.[1] This is hardly surprising; a quarter of a century has elapsed since its launch and like all human endeavours, including medicine itself, it will need to evolve. In the case of EBM those reforms might be summarised in the phrases "medicine is about more than EBM" and "EBM must be about more than medicines".

Medicine is about more than EBM

Healthcare and medicine have undergone reforms at an unprecedented rate during the past three decades. For most of that time the launch of EBM, its evolution as a provider of comparative research and debate about its role have been major preoccupations on the health agenda. As a result the focus of its mission and campaign has also tended to dominate debate. Like all successful campaigns, the EBM movement's carefully focused and restricted mission has been critical. The efficacy and safety of treatments have come under much closer scrutiny as a result of its efforts and the practices of the pharmaceutical industry have been successfully challenged. These have been important contributions to healthcare. However, medicine is about much more than this and the sheer success of the EBM movement in capturing the health agenda coupled with its restricted mission have also distracted attention from the many other areas of concern in medicine, which are in need of scrutiny. In addition, medical professionalism consists of a range of values, all of which are important. Some it seems to me may have received insufficient attention in our efforts to comply with the demands of EBM. These are areas where EBM will need to evolve as it finds its rightful long term place in medicine in the future.

EBM and Conflicting Professional Values

Recommendations for the use of the anti-viral drug, Tamiflu, to prevent influenza was a well-publicised example of conflicting professional values exposed by efforts to pursue EBM, as discussed in Chapter 5. In essence, the dispute centred on an attempt by UK public health physicians to pursue what they considered to be EBM by urging general practitioners (GPs) to prescribe antiviral drugs to elderly people including those in residential care. They hoped in this way to prevent cases of influenza, and thereby to limit spread of the epidemic. The GPs objected on the basis that this might be counter to their obligation to act in the best interest of their patients, believing that some might be harmed by it. Both were acting on the basis of professional values. However, the recommendation to prescribe antiviral drugs for flu prevention was based on a view of EBM as if it were an over-riding value, but which in reality conflicted with other aspects of medical professionalism.

That this should have occurred is hardly surprising given the impact of the EBM movement and its restricted mission. The objection by GPs was correct and in line with legal and regulatory advice and it was also an important first step in correcting misconceptions about the role of EBM in clinical practice. Neither is it surprising that this dispute continues. As I write, the UK Chief Medical Officer has requested the Academy of Medical Science to investigate and provide an independent report on the safety and efficacy of Statins and anti-influenza drugs.[2] The ostensible remit of the Academy's enquiry concerned the reliability of the clinical trials which were used to determine the best evidence on which to base the use of these drugs. However, this dispute also reflects deeper questions about the role of EBM in medicine and its relationship with other values of medical professionalism.

In her letter to the Academy, the Chief Medical Officer was quoted as requesting the report because "there seems to be a view that doctors over-medicate, so it is difficult to trust them, and that clinical scientists are all beset with conflicts of interest from industry funding and are therefore untrustworthy too".[2] The Academy went ahead and set up its enquiry. In response, members of the EBM movement questioned the Academy's ability to act independently, claiming that "medicine is broken" and arguing that medical science is riven with conflicts of interest, and that randomised controlled trials are often regarded as "an unwelcome challenge to medical authority".[3] It would be foolish to argue that medicine is a perfect institution, that doctors are free from potential conflicts of interest or that its institutions can avoid review and reform. They are as liable to these as any other human institution, on the other hand repeated opinion polls have shown that doctors are the most trusted profession in our society.[4] This promotion of the idea that medicine and medical science are untrustworthy rehearses the early rhetoric of the EBM movement,[5] which was successful in launching its campaign and in capturing a patch of moral high ground for its advocacy. More importantly, however, it also contributed to the notion that EBM holds an over-riding place in the set of values that make up medical professionalism. That this should lead to conflict was inevitable. The Tamiflu controversy is an example of this, when efforts to promote a public health interpretation of EBM clashed with GPs views of its likely impact on the professional values they must uphold in dealing with individual patients. The Academy's enquiry as it was commissioned will provide further opinion on the quality and reliability of the research used to establish the safety and efficacy of Tamiflu. This may have added benefit in settling conflicting opinion regarding the relative value of qualitative and quantitative research and how to deal with cases when evidence exists, but is not available to assessors. However, this will not address the professional basis on which the controversy arose and the place of EBM in the overall context of medicine. Thus, whatever the outcome of the enquiry this issue is likely to remain unresolved by it.

EBM therefore still needs to establish its long term place in medicine. While its role in synthesising and prioritising available evidence has been of great benefit, its impact on clinical medicine has not always been so, and as this has grown it has become more apparent, including to the movement itself, which is now calling for a renaissance.[1] Many criticisms have emerged as discussed in Chapter 7, but the most important relate to the role of EBM in the context of individual patient care. Its oversimplified view of evidence failed to recognise the complexities and uncertainties which always attend the care of individuals, encouraged a rule-following and box ticking approach at the expense of judgement and failed to recognise the importance of multimorbidity. There is every reason to hope that EBM will continue to evolve, that these difficulties will be resolved and that EBM will find its long term place within medical professionalism.

EBM Must be about more than Medicines

Caring for patients involves a great deal more than the drugs used to treat them. Inadequate communication and lack of respect were the most frequently cited reasons for complaints to the UK General Medical Council in 2012.[6] Furthermore, everything from the environment in which care is given to staffing levels, organisation and management have an important effect on patients experience of the care they receive. For example the way in which ward rounds are managed will have a major impact on the quality of interaction and communication which patients receive. It is recognised that modern medicine often requires different specialty teams to deal with complex cases and efforts to improve efficiency have resulted in the introduction of shift systems which mean that patients see a different team of doctors from day to day. Such changes can degrade the quality of communication and care patients experience,[7] as will staff levels and the distribution of patients in a busy hospital. All of these have been in a state of unprecedented change with numerous reforms during the past three decades, as discussed in Chapter 4, in attempts to improve healthcare productivity. Despite the enormous upheaval these involve they have been carried out in a virtual vacuum of evidence or timely economic evaluation[8] and may have resulted in high levels of waste.[9,10] Apart from the loss of resources this causes, it also leads to an almost farcical sense of how the NHS is managed and the "basket case" view of the health service, popular in some of the media,[11] but it also impacts directly on the quality of medical care patients receive. The Francis report for example into the failings in medical care at Mid Staffordshire pinpointed poor management, organisation and inadequate staffing levels as being responsible.[12] In the face of reforms based on ideology rather than evidence and an almost "haphazard" approach to policy-making,[13] often with serious adverse consequences,[14] the silence of EBM is striking.

It must surely be ironic that EBM has failed to make any effort to bring evidence to bear on these issues. There may be several reasons for this. EBM originated in an activist movement with a specific mission to campaign for changes in clinical medicine. Like all campaigns its vision was limited and in the case of EBM in two important respects. First, its concept of evidence was restricted to clinical trials. This in effect meant that it could only have an impact on issues related to them, excluding almost everything other than medical treatment. Second, EBM in practice is based on systematic reviews, many of which are commissioned and all require funding. The EBM movement has been at pains to avoid conflicts of interest by declining funding from commercial sources. However, its dependence on commissions and funding may also have contributed to its restricted mission and failure to embrace other important areas of evidence related to medicine. In its present configuration therefore EBM is too restricted in its approach to what evidence matters to medicine and to the care of patients. It also appears to lack sufficient independence to be able to select and scrutinise evidence as it effects medicine and healthcare more widely, particularly in the fields of management and health policy. EBM has been very successful and effective in challenging "medical authority" and the commercial interests of medicine, but much less so in challenging power of governments and health departments and this it seems to me is at the heart of its most significant failure.

Independent EBM

Since its launch, the EBM movement has consistently stated its opposition
to accepting funding from commercial sources that might constitute a conflict of interest. In addition it has presented itself as a challenge to "medical
authority" and to the self-interest of doctors and the medical profession.
These have been important in establishing a degree of independence and a
powerful voice on the relationship between the pharmaceutical industry and
healthcare and also in contributing to the debate on the future place of the
medical profession in society. What it has not done is to put itself in a position of independence from health providers. Thus, it accepts funding from
government departments, not-for-profit insurance, companies and health
management organisations, which have been the most active and powerful
forces for change and reform in healthcare during the past three decades.
Failure of the EBM movement to seek or scrutinise evidence related to these
activities, which have been unprecedented in their range and scope, has been
a serious omission; particularly so when they may be having adverse effects
on the care received by those most in need.[15] And this coupled with its
reliance on these funders for support undermines its claims to independence.
Of course, all organisations constructively involved in healthcare must work
collaboratively and with a degree of interdependence and trust with other
stakeholders and therefore a true state of independence is not possible.
Nevertheless, the present links between the EBM movement and its funders
and its failure to seek or question evidence related to their activities is not
consistent with an independent approach to EBM.

In its report on medical professionalism, the Royal College of Physicians
acknowledged the need that doctors must adapt to changes in the way
healthcare is delivered and to the needs and expectations of patients.[16] However, it also clarified that professionals engaged in healthcare must abide by a
covenant of trust with patients and a moral contract with society, putting
their duty to patients first before all other interests. Consequently they must
be constructive advocates for high quality healthcare based on reliable evidence and be willing to challenge to those who hold political power.[16] It is
clear then that medicine is not just about the treatment which individual
patients receive; it must also embrace the quality of care available to treat
them. It follows that evidence which is relevant to medicine cannot be

confined to drugs and medical devices. The campaign by the EBM movement for high quality research and greater transparency of clinical trials has been of undoubted benefit. However, the amount and quality of evidence on which health service policy in the UK is based is vanishing small or entirely absent[13] in contrast to that required to licence new drugs. The silence of EBM on the former is not consistent with *EBM* in a meaningful sense. Furthermore, the almost ubiquitous presence of EBM in its present configuration and the space given to its various campaigns, however laudable, may be distracting attention from areas in even greater need of scrutiny and reliable evidence. EBM must be more than just a "best buy" for drugs and surgical devices, or a medical version of "Which Magazine". It needs to evolve into an independent movement willing to tackle the evidence base (or lack of it) that is relevant to healthcare more widely and particularly those areas where it is absent.

EBM and Medical Science

EBM is a system for evaluating existing knowledge. It depends on others undertaking original research to develop new knowledge. Unlike EBM which uses systematic approaches to filter and synthesise what is known, science seeks to explore what is unknown. Medicine is of course about much more than science but it has benefited greatly from it and that success depends on a powerful two way relationship between the two. Advances in science have underpinned many of the great strides made in medicine in modern era and the way in which medicine is practiced has had a major influence on the problems tackled by science and how they can benefit patients. A commitment to science and advancing knowledge therefore continues to be an abiding value of medicine. The emergence of EBM has had significant effects on medical science for several reasons.

EBM Replacing Clinical Science

The launch of EBM coincided with a major reallocation of funding for medical research in the UK (discussed in Chapter 4) in 1988 when a version of the customer–provider principal was reintroduced,[17] having previously been rejected for almost all other branches of science. The resulting transfer of research funding to the Department of Health led to a great expansion of health related research aimed at improving healthcare delivery. The EBM movement was a significant beneficiary of this change resulting in its rapid expansion. At the same time, clinical science began to decline as funding was withdrawn,[18] the change being most obvious in the reduction in the numbers of academic clinical posts[19] and fall in research output.[20] It must also be said that members of the EBM movement lobbied against medical science, particularly its much heralded icon Archie Cochrane who claimed that clinical science made no contribution to medical progress (p. 12),[21] was wasteful (p. 44),[21] and should be replaced by comparative research (p. 81).[21] This has continued, and as NHS support for science within the clinical environment has degraded, universities, faced with competitive research assessments, have also withdrawn funding for clinical academic posts in favour of laboratory research, most recently, as I write, at the University Hospital of Wales.[22]

At the centre of this change has been a conflation of the meaning of "research" and "science".[23] This leads to the notion that anything that involves "research" means advancing science and therefore that "health related research" is just another form of science. While it may include some support for original science, most health related research is conducted in order to support and improve delivery of the health service and the comparative research undertaken by the EBM movement is an example of this. It synthesises and summarises existing knowledge rather than seeking to discover new knowledge. This is undoubtedly a valuable service to medicine and to healthcare, but at present its cost effectiveness remains to be examined in significant detail, however, few would dispute its potential value. Nevertheless, it is not and should not be confused with original science, which provides a separate and different function. The decline in clinical science in recent decades has been a major contributing factor to our failure to adapt advances in science for the benefit of patients, now known as the translation gap. An even more serious consequence is our failure even to consider the possibilities that original science can bring to such problems as antimicrobial resistance, preferring instead to focus on making the best of what we have now.[24] This reversal of the great strides made in the early 20th century to introduce science into clinical settings (discussed in Chapter 4), and its retreat back to the laboratory is surely one of the great tragedies to befall medicine in the UK in recent decades. Commitments to science and new knowledge are values intrinsic to medicine because they are essential to maintaining progress and standards of excellence and the decline of recent decades has been harmful to both. Sooner or later the failures which these have caused will demand a rethink as they did at the beginning of the 20th century. That will require much greater clarification of research in terms of its objectives and purpose; drawing a clear distinction between original scientific enquiries on the one hand and research that evaluates what is already known. The simplest solution would be to acknowledge this and fund research accordingly; research aimed at improving healthcare efficiency and productivity including EBM could be funded from the savings it brings and the science budget returned to further science as originally intended. There seems little appetite for this at present; nevertheless, revival of curiosity and the hunger for new knowledge are as inevitable as they are intrinsic to humans.

EBM and the Language of Medicine

Effective use of language was important to the success of the EBM movement and it has proved itself highly effective in its use. Claiming the phrase "EBM" for the name of its campaign was itself a highly successful move. Immediately disarming, and to my knowledge no one has yet come out in support of non-EBM, while at the same time promising something new as if everything which happened before was suspect. And of course it was a wonderful headline. Some years after its launch, in response to criticisms of its promotion of the concept of a hierarchy of evidence (discussed in Chapter 5), a new definition was put forward, which backed away from its early rhetoric; "EBM is the conscientious, judicious and explicit use of current best evidence in making decisions about the care of individual patients".[25] Again, it sounds wonderful, but in reality is so vague as to be almost meaningless (what is best evidence?). However, as one commentator noted what it does is to claim some moral high ground for the movement and disarms its opponents who would presumably have to favour practicing medicine unconscientiously and injudiciously using worse evidence.[26] Rhetoric is important in all communication, but perhaps more so for activist movements and campaigns committed to beliefs or missions. The skilful use of rhetoric, in which the EBM movement excelled, can be powerful in gaining traction for ideas and concepts. However, there is a danger that over reliance on rhetoric and particularly when it is seen to be successful may encourage shifting the nature of debate away from rational analysis in favour of advocacy, campaigns and lobbying. There is some evidence to suggest that this has happened in medicine, particularly in the UK. For example since 2000, the BMJ and Lancet have published 148 and 32 articles respectively with the word "campaign" in the title compared with 8 in the New England Journal of Medicine, and 3 in The Journal of the American Medical Association. As I have previously acknowledged, activism and campaigns can be useful in healthcare and are recognised as legitimate and important means to improve health, particularly public health.[27] Problems may arise however, when the desire to get the message over, relies too heavily on the use of rhetoric which risks degrading debate to a challenge of sound bites on the basis that "if it sounds good it must be good".

Overdiagnosis: Conceals more than it Reveals

Overdiagnosis is a new movement with links to EBM. It is one of several campaigns currently active in healthcare and is a striking example of the power of language and rhetoric in medicine. There has long been concern and debate in medicine that diagnostic tests, particularly screening for breast[28] and prostate cancer[29] can result in some people diagnosed who do not have these conditions and others who receive treatment which is either harmful or gives no benefit (discussed in greater detail in Chapter 7). However, as an issue of concern in medicine it has grown in interest and importance at an extraordinary rate in the past few years and it has received extensive coverage in the medical literature. The BMJ has published a series on the subject around its campaign "Too much Medicine"[30] and it has been the subject of two sell-out international conferences in 2013 and 2014 with a further planned for 2015. It is now regarded as one of several health related movements with which it has overlapping interests, such as EBM, health policy, health economics and health quality and safety.[31] The UK Royal College of GPs has recently setup a standing committee on overdiagnosis with the aim of helping GPs to reduce it. What is remarkable about this increase in the interest and activity related to overdiagnosis is the extraordinary rate with which it rose on the medical agenda. This cannot be attributed to the emergence of some profound new knowledge on the subject; the basic principles are well established based on epidemiological research, and neither can the disagreements and controversy concerning the scientific evidence account for its rise. Rather it seems to reflect a growing presence of activism, campaigns and rhetoric in healthcare discourses. For example medical journals are now more interested in promoting campaigns of various kinds, including on overdiagnosis and much of what is published is authored by editors or journalists, who may even be engaged in supporting the campaign,[32] rather than experts in the field. Indeed many aspects of this campaign are reminiscent of the launch of EBM. We have the catchy title and its apparent incontrovertibility. Then the simultaneous appearance of many articles, publications and conferences dedicated to the subject and the successful recruitment of volunteer advocates. Overdiagnosis is undoubtedly an important matter and needs to be addressed, and those who take a special interest in it have good reason to be concerned. Activism must seem a very useful way to raise awareness of it and the initial success of this campaign must give hope to those involved. Despite these potential benefits, campaigns can also have significant disadvantages.

Distortion of Meaning

The term overdiagnosis means an excess of diagnoses; too many people are being given a particular diagnosis. It arises from epidemiological methods which can provide important information about the health of populations based on a yes or no answer as to whether a particular diagnosis has been made. The term overdiagnosis then is essentially a term of quantity based on the idea of diagnosis as a binary function in medicine. You either have it or you don't. While this can be useful in public health research, if used in the context of clinical medicine it distorts the meaning of diagnosis in several important ways. First, diagnosing a patient's illness is far more complicated than a simple yes or no. A full diagnosis should include (i) the nature of the illness, (ii) its rate of progression, (iii) the stage it has reached, (iv) what has caused it, (v) what complications have occurred and (vi) the likely prognosis. This matters not only because the overdiagnosis is misleading in terms of language, but also because it distorts how we should think about the problem, and how it might be mitigated. The idea of overdiagnosis as simply too many diagnoses suggests that the answer is to make fewer of them and this is reinforced when the concept is linked to another campaign with a similar message such as "Too Much Medicine".[30] But in reality, if too many or indeed too few people are given a particular diagnosis and are receiving too much or too little treatment, the problem underlying it may be one of several. The diagnosis may simply be wrong, or it might be inadequate if, for example, the stage of the illness or the rate of progression have not been clarified. Alternatively the diagnosis may have been based on a test which is unreliable. Each of these is important in finding solutions, but all are masked by the rhetoric of overdiagnosis, which reduces the problem to one of "too much", and the solution to "do less".

Take for example the problem of overdiagnosis of prostate cancer. The background to this is the relative inaccuracy of the Prostate Specific Antigen (PSA) test. At present, the evidence indicates that if PSA testing is used to screen men for prostate cancer it can save lives, however, this benefit is offset by the fact that it also gives positive results in some men leading to unnecessary or harmful surgery.[33] PSA testing therefore needs to be considered with caution until this is resolved. The implication of the "overdiagnosis" and "too much medicine" campaigns is that we should diagnose fewer patients by testing fewer people for (PSA) levels. The problem with this "do less" approach is that it grossly oversimplifies a serious medical challenge. It belies the reality that prostate cancer is the most common malignancy in men and a major cause of cancer deaths, it obscures the causes of the problem and distracts from what is needed to resolve them. The main cause is of course our reliance on the PSA test, which has been with us for over half a century and is well known to be woefully inaccurate. It results in inaccurate, incomplete or plain wrong diagnoses in too many people. So the problem then is not overdiagnosis, but incorrect diagnoses and the consequences are not only over-treatment, but also failure to detect many cancers and many men dying from undetected disease. The obvious and urgent need is for more accurate tests, to be able to diagnose prostate cancer with greater precision, to offer patients more appropriate treatment and ultimately to save more lives.

The selection of "overdiagnosis" and "overtreatment" for the purposes of activism and campaigning on a problem such as prostate cancer obscures its real complexity and distracts attention from what is needed to make progress. They are newly invented terms conveying the idea of something novel and original, but in reality they mislead the search for durable solutions. In that sense they are representative of the increasing use of rhetoric in dealing with health issues during the past two decades. This oversimplification also tends to degrade the quality of discourse. For example one commentator described overdiagnosis as a science[34] while another warned that a definition of it has not yet even been agreed and that it might need one definition for the purposes of advocacy and another for research purposes,[31] as if like Humpty Dumpty, it could mean what we chose it to mean. This rhetoric also suggests that overtreatment is intrinsic to prostate cancer and other illnesses and the notion that as more patients are treated more are harmed. The answer then is to do less. But the limitations of the PSA test are a problem today; understanding of the disease is advancing rapidly and there is every reason to expect that better tests will become available in the future. That should greatly reduce the incidence of false positive results and allow more precise treatment. But the rates of diagnosis and treatment might not change and could possibly increase if better diagnostics detect more cases with greater accuracy. The objective of good medicine should be to reduce unnecessary or harmful treatment as far as possible, but at the same time to find better ways to offer appropriate treatment to all of those who need it, including patients dying today due to lack of adequate care. Nothing of this complexity is captured in the simplified rhetoric of campaigns such as "overdiagnosis" and "overtreatment". Indeed, it is so vague and yet sounds so plausible, it becomes a useful rhetorical device for other advocacy that may have adverse unintended consequences for the care of patients. For example, "overdiagnosis" is suggested as an economic target for "reducing waste" in the UK health service.[35] But without considering the wider needs for improving outcomes for conditions such as prostate and breast cancer, campaigns to "do less" risk undermining progress needed to deal with the challenges they pose. This is especially so in the UK which has higher a mortality from cancers than most western countries.[36]

Activism has a long history in efforts to improve public health. Some have made important contributions, for example in the case of tobacco, others less so. Success depends on a mix of science, politics, media engagement, timing and perhaps luck.[27] The narrow focus of all campaigns means that they lack objectivity in relation to overall priorities. This risks marginalising important and related issues, for example the HIV/AIDS campaign made a major contribution to securing increased availability of antiretroviral drugs for millions of people in poorer countries, but its success also distracted attention from the need to establish the basic healthcare systems needed to manage treatment and from the need to deal with other important factors involved in the spread of HIV/AIDS, such as poverty, lack of education and individual powerlessness.[37] In contrast to the history of activism in health, the flurry of campaigns in recent years, have focused more on the healthcare system itself. Campaigns such as "Too much medicine" and "Overdiagnosis" address important issues. But while strong on rhetoric they are weak in terms of EBM. While they have the backing of good science showing that some patients receive treatment that is unhelpful or harmful, no attempt is made to consider any evidence about its causes or what remedy is needed to resolve them. Rather it seems as if the advocated remedy, "do less", is the object of the campaign and the evidence chosen to fit it. But this selective approach to evidence is not consistent with any meaningful understanding of EBM.

It seems ironic that such campaigns should be linked to EBM, but then the EBM movement itself began as a campaign and with a strong use of rhetoric and its success may well have been an encouragement to others. In contrast its advocacy has always been for rational analysis of evidence. Its future must surely be in this direction; EBM cannot be just another lobbying activity or indeed a movement. It needs to be imbedded as a value of integrity within medicine, objective and unbiased both in its selection of evidence and its analysis of it. There needs to be a clear distinction between advocacy and EBM. All campaigns are a form of lobbying; whether we agree or disagree with their objectives or how worthy they may be and irrespective of whether their advocates claim to be representatives of or practitioners of EBM, this is not EBM and linking such activities to EBM devalues it. This seems to me to be critical for the future of EBM.

I have no doubt that the principles of EBM will remain an important value in medicine. They are already recognised within the system of medical professionalism. EBM must evolve to be applied in the context of other values and obligations in that system (Box 9.1). It must be independent and

---

Box 9.1   The Future of EBM.

1. A recognised value in medical professionalism.
2. Applied in the context of other values and obligations in medicine.
3. Independent and unbiased in its selection and analysis of evidence.
4. Applicable to all aspects of medicine.
5. Based on objective and rational analysis of evidence.

unbiased both in the selection of evidence it is applied to. And it must be applicable to all evidence related to medicine and healthcare. It must be objective and rational in its analysis of evidence.

Conclusions

Efforts to ensure medicine is based on reliable evidence have a long history, but the launch of EBM in the 1990s gave it a new impetus and led to it becoming embedded as a recognised value of medical professionalism. The principles of EBM concern rational evaluation of evidence. In contrast its launch, which proved extremely successful, relied heavily on advocacy and rhetoric and was focused almost exclusively on medicines and medical devices. In the initial configuration of EBM it was proposed that evidence derived from clinical trials was of greater value and importance than other forms of evidence related to medical care. Although this position has since been abandoned it has led to conflicts of professional values when clinicians were urged to treat patients on the basis of trial based EBM, but which they believed conflicted with their wider obligations to patients. Some ambiguity may remain, however, reviews of medical professionalism and the regulation of doctors now recognise EBM as a value doctors should uphold as part of and in the context of their overall commitments and obligations.

The restriction of EBM to evidence related to drugs and medical devices has left great swathes of evidence concerning healthcare untouched, most notably, the reforms of healthcare delivery and reconfiguration of its management. This has to change if EBM is to be a meaningful value in medicine. EBM must be and be seen to be independent both in the selection of evidence it is applied to as well as in analysing it. It must also be concerned with evidence related to all aspects of healthcare or the lack of evidence. EBM embodies a set of principles that are widely applicable in medicine; it cannot at the same time be a campaign restricted to a preconceived mission. Indeed practitioners of EBM should be wary of all campaigns, since they invariably select evidence to fit their objectives. Despite its successful use of rhetoric and advocacy for its launch, EBM must be more than just another lobbying activity. It has shone a bright light on important areas of medical practice, but if it is to have a meaningful and durable future as a set of principles in medicine, it must begin to illuminate the many areas in medicine and healthcare that operate in the shadows of evidence.

References

1. Greenhalgh T, Howick J, Maskrey N (2014). Evidence-Based Medicine: A Movement in Crisis? *BMJ*, 348, g3725.
2. Wise J (2015), CMO asks for Review of Drug Evaluation in Wake of Controversy Over Statins. *BMJ*, 350, h3300.
3. Goldacre B, Heneghan, C (2015). How Medicine is Broken and How to Fix it. *BMJ*, 350, h3397.
4. Polls and Publications. Ipsos MORI. Available at: https://www.ipsos-mori.com/ researchpublications/researcharchive/3504/Politicians-trusted-less-than-estate-agents-bankers-and-journalists.aspx (Accessed on 1/7/2015).
5. Blythe M, Cochrane A (1989). *One Man's Medicine: An Autobiography of Professor Archie Cochrane.* London: *BMJ* Publishing.
6. General Medical Council. The State of Medical Education and Practice in the UK. Available at: http://www.gmc-uk.org/publications/somep2012.asp?WT.ac= WBPR120918 (Accessed on 9/7/2-15).
7. Ward Rounds in Medicine: Principles for Best Practice. A Joint Publication of the Royal College of Physicians and Royal College of Nursing. Available at: https://www.rcplondon.ac.uk/sites/default/files/documents/ward-rounds-in-medicine-web.pdf (Accessed on 9/7/2015).
8. Walshe K (2014). Counting the Cost of Lansley's NHS Reorganisation. *BMJ*, 349, g6340.
9. National Audit Office (2013). Department of Health: Managing the Transition to the Reformed Health System. Available at: https://www.nao.org.uk/report/ managing-the-transition-to-the-reformed-health-system-2/ (Accessed on 11/12/2015).
10. Clough C. Final Report: Independent Review of Nottingham Dermatology Services. Available at: http://bit.ly/1IARWyg (Accessed on 12/7/2015).
11. Chorley M (2014). "Unintelligible Gobbledygook" of NHS Reforms were our Biggest Mistake in Government, Senior Tories admit. Available at: Daily Mail. www. dailymail.co.uk/news/article-2790785/unintelligible-gobbledygook-nhs-reforms-biggest-mistake-governmentsenior-tories-admit.html. (Accessed on 11/12/2015).
12. Department of Health (2010). Independent Inquiry into care Provided by Mid Staffordshire NHS Foundation Trust January 2005 — March 2009. Chaired by Robert Francis QC. Available at: http://www.dh.gov.uk/en/Publicationsand statistics/Publications/PublicationsPolicyAndGuidance/DH_113018 (Accessed on 9/7/2015).
13. The NHS (2005): A National Health Sham. *Lancet*, 366, 1239.
14. Clough C. Final Report: Independent Review of Nottingham Dermatology Services. 4 Jun 2015. Available at: http://bit.ly/1IARWyg (Accessed on 11/12/2015).

15. Mannion R, Davies HTO (2005). Taking Stock of Social Capital in the Production of Health Care. *J Health Serv Res Policy*,10, 129–130.
16. Doctors in Society Medical Professionalism in a Changing World (2005). *Report of a Working Party*, London: Royal College of Physicians.
17. House of Lords Select Committee on Science and Technology (1987–1988). *Priorities in Medical Research, 3rd Report Session*. London: HMSO.
18. Sheridan DJ (2012). *The Rise and Fall of Medical Science in the 20ᵗʰ Century*. *In* Medical Science in the 21st Century: Sunset or New dawn? London: Imperial College Press.
19. Johnston K. Cuts Force UK Universities into "Glamorous" Medical Research. *Nature*, 1987, 327, 262.
20. Smith R (1888). International Comparisons of Funding and Output Research: Bye Bye Britain. *BMJ*, 296, 409–412.
21. Cochrane AL (1972). *Effectiveness and Efficiency: Random Reflections on Health Services*, 2nd Ed. London: Nuffield Provincial Trust, pp. 12, 44, 81, 83.
22. More than 60 Academic Jobs Reportedly under Threat at Cardiff University's School of Medicine. WalesOnline. Available at: http://www.walesonline.co.uk/news/health/more-60-academic-jobs-reportedly-9307138 (Accessed on 12/7/2015).
23. Sheridan DJ (2012). *Advances in Medicine: How are they made?* *In* Medical Science in the 21ˢᵗ Century; Sunset or New dawn? London: Imperial College Press.
24. Tonkin-Crine S, Walker AS, Butler CC (2015). Contribution of Behavior Science to Antibiotic Stewardship. *BMJ*, 350, h3413.
25. Sackett DL, Rosenberg WC, Gray JAM (1996). Evidence-Based Medicine: What it is and What it isn't. *BMJ*, 312, 71–72.
26. Greenhalgh T (2012). Why do We Always End Up Here? Evidence-Based Medicine's Conceptual *cul-de-sacs* and some Off-road Alternative Routes. *J Prim Health Care*, 4(2), 92–97.
27. Berridge V (2007). Public Health Activism. *BMJ*, 335, 1310–1312.
28. Fox MS (1979). On the Diagnosis and Treatment of Breast Cancer. *JAMA*, 241, 489–494.
29. Etzioni R1, Penson DF, Legler JM, di Tommaso D, Boer R, Gann PH, Feuer EJ (2002). Overdiagnosis due to Prostate-Specific Antigen Screening: Lessons from US Prostate Cancer Incidence Trends. *J Natl Cancer Inst*, 94, 981–990.
30. Too much Medicine. *BMJ*, Available at: http://www.bmj.com/too-much-medicine (Accessed on 16/7/2015).
31. Carter SM, Rogers W, Heath I, Degeling C, Doust J, Barratt A (2015). The Challenge of Overdiagnosis Begins with its Definition. *BMJ*, 350, h869.

32. Moynahan R (2015). Preventing Overdiagnosis: The myth, the Music and the Medical Meeting. *BMJ*, 350, h1370.
33. Attard G, Parker C, Eeles RA, Schröder F, Tomlins SA, Tannock I, Drake CG, de Bono JS (2015). Prostate cancer. *Lancet*, Available at http://dx.doi.org/10.1016/S0140–6736(14)61947–4 (Accessed on 11/12/2015).
34. Moynihan R (2013). Science of Overdiagnosis to be Served up with a Good Dose of Humility. *BMJ*, 347, f5157.
35. Better Value in the NHS The role of Changes in Clinical Practice. The King's, Fund. Available at: www.kingsfund.org.uk/sites/files/kf/field/field_document/better-value-nhs-summary-July-2015.pdf (Accessed on 20/7/2015).
36. International Comparisons of Healthcare Quality. Nuffield Trust. Available at: http://www.qualitywatch.org.uk/international (Accessed on 11/12/2015).
37. Gomo E, Mate R, Mugurungi O, Magure T, Campbell B, Dehne K, Halperin D. (2011). Local Perceptions of Forms, Timing and Causes of Behaviour Change in Response to the AIDS Epidemic in Zimbabwe. *AIDS behav*, 15, 487–498.

Index

A

Activism, 15, 31, 52, 144, 206–210
Advocacy in Healthcare, 22, 25, 48,
  146, 154, 156, 158, 161, 174,
  183–184, 187, 191–192, 199,
  206–210
Alanson, Edward, 10
Antibiotic Resistance, 32, 135–140
Authority, 4, 8–9, 13, 61, 79, 113,
  120, 174, 179, 199, 201

B

Biomedical Literature, 7–8
Black, Douglas, 73–74
Brand, 1–2, 152, 162, 166–167

C

Campaign in Healthcare, 48, 50–52,
  144, 153–158, 160–161, 177–179,
  205–209
Cardiac Arrhythmia Suppression Trial
  (CAST), 115–118
Certainty, 95–97

Chain, Ernst, 135, 138
Cheselden, William, 11–12
Cinchona Bark, 10
Clark, John, 10
Clifton, Francis, 9
Clinical Epidemiology, 4, 6, 9, 14
Clinical Experience, 4, 6, 8, 23–24, 28,
  53, 96–97, 104–107, 110, 128–129,
  138–139, 144, 146, 151, 166, 183
  mechanical rules in [see under
    mechanical rules]
  reasoning in [see under reasoning]
Clinical Guidelines, 107–110, 120,
  153–158, 164, 184, 186
Clinical Judgement, 103–108,
  110–114, 118, 120–121, 161, 176,
  183–187, 190
  mechanical rules in [see under
    mechanical rules]
  reasoning in [see under reasoning]
Cochrane Collaboration, 37–58
Cochrane Collaboration and
  comparative research, 42, 49
  efficiency, 43

funding, 37–40, 50, 83, 88
future challenges, 41
mission, 39–43
Nuffield Trust, 37
sponsorship, 39
volunteers, 37, 39
waste, 50–52
Cochrane Library, 38–39, 153
Cochrane, Archie, 21–32
Comparative Research, 39, 49–53, 84, 86, 88, 104, 112, 118, 125–127
Coronary Care Units, 27–30
Crimean War, 13
Critical Appraisal, 5, 7
Currie, Jacque, 126
Currie, Pierre, 126

D

Dainton, Frederick, 71–73
Report, 71
Darwin, Erasmus, 12
Diagnostic Criteria, 30, 108–110, 185
Digoxin, 12

E

East India Company, 10
EBM
achievements, 153
advocacy and, 22, 25, 48, 146, 154, 156, 158, 161, 174, 183–184, 187, 191–192, 199, 206–210
campaigns and, 158–159
clinical guidelines and, 154–157
clinical practice, impact on, 151–167, 198
conflicts of interest, 43, 199, 201
definition, 2, 44, 205, 209
future of, 197–210

history of, 3, 9, 14, 19, 38, 45, 60, 152, 197
in crisis, 161, 165, 167
independence of, 202
limitations of, 161–164
medical professionalism and, 173–193, 198
medical science and, 125–147, 154, 173, 203–204
myth making rhetoric, 103–104, 130
National Health Research Authority, 79–84
NICE and, 156
origins, 1
overdiagnosis and, 159
sponsorship, 1, 39
working group, 4
Edler, Inge, 127
Evidence
best, 2, 99, 152, 199, 205
hierarchy of, 5–8, 15, 97–103, 105, 110–113, 119, 134–135, 144, 176, 183, 192, 205
interpretation of, 98–103, 105, 109, 113, 120, 199
Expert Opinion, 111–112

F

Fleming, Alexander, 135, 142, 144, 163
Fletcher, Walter Morley, 62–63, 65
Florey, Howard, 135–140, 142, 145
Foxglove, 12

H

Haldane, Viscount, 60–62
MRC, 62–63
principal, 60–61

report, 60–61
Rothschild report, 61, 71
Health Related Research, 30–33, 45, 59–88, 154, 204
Health Services Research, 75, 77–78
Hertz, Carl Helmuth, 127
Holland, Walter, 68, 81
House of Lords Committee on Science and Technology 1988, 76, 78–79
Hunter, John, 10

I

Index Medicus, 2

J

Jones, Duckett, 109

K

Knowledge, 2, 18, 49–53, 64–65, 86, 95–91, 101, 105–106, 151, 163, 173–175, 180, 182–184, 203

L

Lewis, Thomas, 64
Lind, James, 12, 41

M

Maclean, Charles, 13
McMaster Model, 3–6, 8–9, 14, 37, 45, 84–85
McMaster PLUS, 45
Mechanical Rules, 105, 110, 119–120
Medical Professionalism
charter for the New Millennium, 173, 191
clinical guidelines and, 184
evidence and, 183
failures of, 174–175

General Medical Council and, 181–182
George Bernard Shaw and, 175
healthcare management and, 177–178, 185, 188
judgement and, 183
leadership and, 187–190
NICE and, 188
Royal College of Physicians and, 178
values of, 176, 178–181
Medical Science, 27, 52–53, 60, 65, 88, 125–147, 154, 203
certainty in [see under certainty]
clinical practice and, 65, 125, 143, 204
history of, 63–89
hypothesis in, 28–29, 51–52, 95, 115–118, 129–134
knowledge in [see under knowledge]
reasoning and, 129–135
research and, 50, 61, 86, 204
uncertainty in [see under uncertainty]

N

National Health Research Authority, 79–80
Nightingale, Florence , 13–14, 131
Nuffield Trust, 25, 37, 39, 60, 67, 168, 177

O

Osler, William, 64, 151–152, 166
Osmond, Paul, 73
report, 73
Overdiagnosis, 153, 159, 161, 206–209

P

Paradigm
   new, 4, 7–8, 14, 97, 177, 183
   shift, 8
Penicillin, 27, 135–138, 142, 144

R

Reasoning, 95–97, 106–107, 110,
   115–120, 129–134, 173, 179,
   183–184
   mechanistic, 110, 115, 117–120,
      136, 144
Roentgen, Wilhelm, 126
Rothschild, Lord, 70–71
   customer–contractor principal,
      70–71
   report, 60–61
   report reversed, 73

S

Scurvy, 12, 41
Snow, John, 130–135
   cholera and, 130–135
   reasoning and, 130–135
   truth and myth, 130

T

Tamiflu, 46–49, 98–100, 198–200
Translation Gap, 65, 143, 204
Trend, Burke, 69–71

U

Uncertainty, 95–97, 160

W

Withering, William, 12–13

Printed in the United States
By Bookmasters